Indoor Epidemic

93% Inside Steals Sleep, Focus & Years--The 7% Outdoor Rx Restores Them

Seven proven outdoor prescriptions to reset your internal clock, think clearer, and sleep deeper

John La Puma, MD

John La Puma, MD

Copyright
© John La Puma. All rights reserved. No part of Indoor Epidemic may be copied, stored, or shared without written permission from the author or publisher.

Disclaimer
This book shares the author's views and ideas. It does not give medical or professional advice. Readers should speak with their own health clinicians before using any methods described in this book. The author and publisher are not responsible for any harm or loss that may occur from the use of the material in this book. Some images in this book were generated using Gamma and Google Gemini. The author does not claim copyright in these AI-generated images.

PAPERBACK ISBN 979-8-9935109-0-3
EBOOK ISBN 979-8-9935109-1-0
HARDCOVER ISBN 979-8-9935109-2-7
JACKET ISBN 979-8-9935109-3-4

Dedication

For Kandi, who makes the world go 'round.

Acknowledgments

Thank you to Wellness Imprints for believing from the start. Special thanks to my publishing team for steady craft and care.

With gratitude to Ioan Hanes, MD, and Ioannis Arkadianos, MD, (ELMO), Susan Benigas, and Beth Frates, MD (ACLM). Mark Silverberg, MD, Alex Soffici, MD, Ron Werft (Santa Barbara Cottage Hospital), and the Cottage Health community, who prove that gardens and genuinely good food belong in health care.

Thank you to Barrett Cordero, Beth Ford, Ken Sperling and Jonathan Wygant (BigSpeak), and Diane Goodman (Goodman Speakers Bureau) for opening doors and believing in this message. And Oprah: thank you for the inspiration.

I'm grateful to early hosts and sponsors: A4M (American Academy of Anti-Aging Medicine); Advocate Aurora Health-Lutheran General Hospital; California Baby with Jessica Soy, CEO and principal sponsor; The Center for Continuing Professional Development (CCPD), David Geffen School of Medicine at UCLA; Division of Lifestyle Medicine, DGSOM at UCLA; and the Ogden Surgical–Medical Society.

For early invitations that helped shape this work: Steven Barag, DO; S. Dominique Del Chiaro, M.Ed. (Senior Manager, Healthy Living, Stanford); Elizabeth Ko, MD, of UCLA; Patty de Vries (Stanford University); Maria Failla; Alex Strauss; Jeff Tkach (Rodale Institute); and Kelcey Trefethen (Ending Burnout).

Thank you to: Sharon Horesh Bergquist, MD; Robert Graham, MD; Uma Naidoo, MD; Drew Ramsey, MD; and Colin Zhu, DO, for building the culinary-medicine bridge in clinical care.

With appreciation to: Susan Abookire, MD; Melissa Lem, MD; Dan Nadeau; Wallace J. Nichols, Ph.D. (in memoriam); James Rippe, MD; Scott Stoll, MD; and Robert Zarr, MD, for leadership, evidence, and courage in making nature a clinical ally.

Thank you to Scott Amyx (Uplifty AI), Bob Barnett, Angela Myers, Kevin Pho, MD, and Mark Sylvester (Coastal Intelligence) for thoughtful coverage and amplification. Social support from Kyler Smigaj helped these ideas reach farther.

I am grateful for the collaboration and craft from Chef Rick Bayless; Dominique Crisp; Chef Vincent Donatelli; Chef Massimo Falsini; Tara Penke; Nik Ramirez; Greg & Daisy Ryan; and Chef John Wayne.

Thank you to: Rachel Callahan (UC ANR Agritourism); Billy & Will Carleton (Las Palmalitas); Steve Clifton (Vega Vineyard & Farm); Richard Dallam, FAIA (Managing Partner, NBBJ) for the opportunity to design healing gardens; Gerri French; Jane Loura; Phil McGrath; Ed Mickleson; Tony Murry; Ana & Jesse Smith (White Buffalo Land Trust); and Noey Turk (native plants). Thanks also to Organic Certifiers and the Real Organic Project for setting a high bar for regenerative practice.

For unwavering support and friendship: Michael DeLapa, Kathy Mackey, Maureen O'Rourke, David Schiedermayer, Richard Salzberg, Leslie Thomas, Steve Tureff, and Thomas Whittemore.

To Drs. Mike and Nancy Roizen: thank you for hosting us. And to Kandi: for your creativity, inspiration, joy, belief and confidence. To your family (Luke and Lindsey, Cindi, Mitzi, Peggy, and nieces Devon and Shannon): you make this work a family endeavor.

Let's keep building.

I look forward to bringing Indoor Epidemic solutions and Outdoor Rx programs to workplaces, schools, media outlets and to more clinicians, campuses and communities worldwide.

Author Bio

Dr. John La Puma, MD, FACP, better known as ChefMD™, is a physician, chef, and author at the forefront of the food-as-medicine and Outdoor Rx movements. A two-time *New York Times* bestselling author, he blends science and storytelling to help you feel younger, think clearer, and live longer and better with dozens of simple, evidence-based outdoor and nutrition tips.

Scan for Exclusive Reader Bonuses

As a thank you for joining the movement toward better health in the Indoor Epidemic era, scan the QR code below to access bonus content created just for you.

What's Inside?

You'll find tools, resources, and insights that expand on the book, plus a few surprises we couldn't fit in print.

Includes access to:

- Practical tools to apply what you've read
- Bonus health trackers and device recommendations
- Reader-only updates from Dr. La Puma
- Special offers and early access to new content

Scan to access Indoor Epidemic Exclusives (Outdoor Rx Cheat Sheet, recommended devices, and simple tools to track your results).

Disclaimer

Indoor Epidemic contains the opinions and ideas of its author. It is not to be considered medical, professional, or personal services. Readers should consult their own health professionals before adopting the suggestions and advice in the book. The author and publisher specifically disclaim all responsibility for any liability, loss, or risk, personal or otherwise, which is incurred as a consequence, directly or indirectly, of the use and application of the contents of this book.

Introduction

This Is Not a Self-Help Book. This Is a Rescue Mission.

You are here because some part of you feels trapped. Your body aches from sitting, your brain fogs from staring at screens, and your spirit feels flattened by the sheer weight of modern life. You've tried the apps, the hacks, and the trendy diets. You've listened to the podcasts and bought the supplements. And yet, you are still running on fumes.

We now recognize this relentless digital consumption, in which we consume more data than our nervous system can metabolize-as Digital Obesity, a biological condition driving chronic anxiety, inflammation, and premature aging.

This book is your field manual for Analog Wellness: an evidence-based longevity upgrade designed to restore what modern life has depleted. **We tap into the analog tools you already own or can easily pick up, like bound or loose-leaf journals, offline clocks and simple trackers to support and strengthen your outdoor reset.** It's not anti-tech; it's pro-balance. A foundational reset that strengthens your body, sharpens your mind, and extends your healthspan (see Glossary), through intentional, science-backed time outdoors.

Here's what your body knows that your mind has forgotten: Every hour you spend sealed inside is an hour your body quietly and prematurely ages. Not just on the surface, but deep within, where your cells are suffering injury and struggling to repair themselves. Your body keeps its own clock and it's falling behind. We're trading long-term vitality for comfort (filtered air, artificial light, glowing screens) that soothes in the moment but gives away years of life, killing us softly, quietly, and indoors.

But the most powerful antidote to premature aging is free. It doesn't come in a pill, a powder, or an app. It's just outside your door, and it may be the most overlooked, lifesaving medicine your body has ever needed.

This book provides the foundational layer for any longevity stack or biohack, especially those that lead to lasting habits. Nature isn't alternative medicine: it's foundational medicine, and it amplifies the effectiveness of supplements, therapy, and optimization.

Benefits of Nature Exposure

- 2 hours/week: noticeable benefits begin
- 3-5 hours/week: peak healthspan gains
- More than 5 hours: benefits plateau but remain

One way I think of nature is as the original lifestyle+ therapy, our oldest, low-tech package for total health and the most accessible.

Decades of research, including a study of 700,000 U.S. veterans, point to one clear truth. Stack deep sleep, real food, daily movement, close bonds, and time in nature, and you can gain up to twenty extra years.

Deliberately layering nature-based practices such as sunrise or sunset walks, green exercise, forest bathing, and soil-to-skin gardening reboots your body's innate resilience.

This is not a self-help book filled with gentle suggestions and vague affirmations. This is a field manual for a rescue mission. Your own.

Our indoor, screen-based lives have become so extreme that even internet slang now begs us to touch grass. This is more than a meme. Two-thirds of Gen Z and more than half of millennials admit they sometimes don't go outside for days at a time. Children today spend half as much time outdoors as their parents did, with a third never playing outside daily. Adults now spend four to six hours a day on recreational screen time.

We are not only fighting this epidemic for ourselves. We are fighting it for our children, who are facing a silent siege. Since schools began handing out pandemic-era digital devices, many students have stopped going outside altogether.

Teachers describe children who no longer play, explore, or move the way they once did. Screens have replaced the natural rhythms that develop attention, curiosity, and emotional regulation.

The consequences are measurable. Between 2016 and 2022, antidepressant prescriptions for children aged 12 to 17 rose by 69 percent. Twenty-two percent of college students now report symptoms of depression.

Digital devices, introduced as early as pre-K, act as digital traps. They override the steady grounding values we try to build as parents and train young brains to seek stimulation that is faster, louder, and harder to escape.

We've taken moments that should feel grounding and turned them into constant stimulation. That's ultra-processed time. It's the time-version of ultra-processed food: addictive, depleted, and hard to stop consuming.

I know some of you dream of quitting your job and moving to a cabin in the woods and, honestly, I respect that impulse. After all, I bought an abandoned nursery. I also know that neither path is realistic for most people.

Here's what is realistic: you're already spending 93% of your time indoors, anyway. That means the 7% you do venture outside needs to work like medicine. The core truth of this book is that real, measurable health is found in micro-doses and micro-practices that work immediately.

That's the heart of the **7% Outdoor Rx,** which we often refer to as **The 7% Solution** (see Glossary). Just five minutes in green space measurably boosts mood, and fifteen minutes of early sun resets your entire biological clock. Every walk to your car becomes a potential nature dose.

Every outdoor lunch break becomes an opportunity to enjoy the pleasures and benefits of nature therapy. Every moment of walking the dog becomes a way to connect. I will teach you to turn those scattered outdoor minutes into concentrated healing.

How to Use This Book

Think of this book as a workbook and mission guide. My goal is to act as your coach translating the science and giving you clear steps to act on right away. There's no filler here, only what works. It's a smart way to use your 7%. Light is your main cue, but food, movement, and social contact are powerful time-setters too. Use them daily to keep your internal clock on track.

Each of the first seven chapters follows a simple structure:

The Why (Your Science Snapshot):

This provides the scientific foundation for each practice. You'll see how your outdoor actions affect your body and why these habits work so well.

The How-To (Your Mission):

Here you'll find step-by-step tools you can use now. Each component includes a clear, specific protocol that fits into any schedule.

Helpful Tips and Bonus Info (Nature Notes & Doctor It Up!):

These sections help you fine-tune your practice. Nature Notes share new research highlights, and Doctor It Up! gives insider tips to boost your results and solve common challenges.

Throughout the book, you'll use Your Outdoor Rx Action Space as your personal log for recording observations and tracking progress. It helps you turn science into lived experience and feel the results of nature's healing power.

Indoor Epidemic

You might think this sounds impossible: city life, work, family, and little free time. Maybe you're caring for someone or stuck indoors all day. This book is written for you. Whether you get outside 7% or 0.7% of your day, it meets you where you are.

This isn't about quitting your job or escaping to the woods. It's about using the nature around you: street trees, a park bench, even a view of the sky as tools for health. The methods here work anywhere because they're based on human biology. You already have what you need to start.

This is your invitation to reclaim focus, energy, and well-being. You already spend time outdoors: nearly 12 hours a week, in small bits. The goal isn't to add more hours, but to turn those scattered moments into true Outdoor Rx. Quality matters more than quantity.

Every bit counts. A greener path-one lined with trees instead of asphalt-can lower your risk of death by about 4%. A simple choice like walking down a leafy street can improve your health and longevity.

That's the heart of The 7% Solution. It's not about living outside. It's about turning a fraction of your existing outdoor time into medicine. Just two hours a week can shift you from the indoor epidemic toward longer, healthier years.

It's time to step outside. You already have The 7% Solution. Let's use it.

Contents

Introduction x
How to Use This Book xiv
Chapter 1: Meeting the Morning Sun: Your Daily Reset Button & Biological Igniter 17
Chapter 2: Sky, Space, and Sea Medicine: How Vastness Heals Your Brain 44
Chapter 3: Forest-Bathing Rx: Inhale Immunity, Reset Your Nervous System 86
Chapter 4: Move Like You Mean It 129
Chapter 5: The Nature Connection: The Outdoors as Medicine for Isolation and Longevity 167
Chapter 6: Gardening Rx: Cultivating Your Longevity from Soil to Plate 201
Chapter 7: Wind Down with Darkness: Your Nightfall Ritual for Deep Rest 241
Chapter 8: Your 7-Day Outdoor Rx Reset Plan 289
Chapter 9: Keeping It Going: Making Your Outdoor Rx Stick 307
Chapter 10: Bonus Practices: Extra Ideas for Deepening Your Analog Wellness 321
Bonus Rx #1: Companion Animal Connection: How Positive Regard Rewires the Brain 325
Bonus Rx #2: Birding: Your Gateway to Wildness 328
Bonus Rx #3: Houseplants: Your Indoor Nature Prescription 331
Bonus Rx #4: Immersion, Adventure & Purposeful Healing 333
Bonus Rx #5: Nature Art & Creative Observation 335
Conclusion: Seriously, You Belong Outside 339
Glossary 344

Chapter 1:
Meeting the Morning Sun: Your Daily Reset Button & Biological Igniter

Introduction:
Your First Mission Against the Indoor Epidemic

This is your first mission. It is the foundational strike in our crusade against the Indoor Epidemic.

The most potent tool for reclaiming your energy, sharpening your focus, and resetting your entire biological operating system costs nothing, requires no special equipment, and is waiting for you just outside your door. I'm talking about morning sunlight.

Beyond setting your Master Clock for energy and focus, daylight also primes your body for Vitamin D synthesis. Morning light readies your receptors, and midday sun (when UVB rays peak) flips the biochemical switch in your skin to produce this essential vitamin. Skipping outdoor light starves your bones, immune system, and even your brain of Vitamin D's ability to protect your DNA and lift your mood. When you get outside light, you're fortifying your body at the molecular level as a form of Outdoor Rx.

I will try to dismantle the myth that you are just not a morning person. I will show you why you feel groggy, unmotivated, and dependent on caffeine to start your day.

> **Watercooler Fact:**
> 86/7/7 Rule: Most people spend 93% of their time indoors-- 86% in buildings and 7% in vehicles--but optimizing your 7% outdoors can revolutionize your health.

The culprit is a severe lack of a specific, required biological signal: the photons from the early morning sun entering your eyes. This is a physiological necessity that our modern lives have stripped away, with devastating consequences for our health, affecting everything from our risk of diabetes and dementia to our too-often daily experience of burnout and anxiety.

I will show you precisely how this light acts as a master switch for your brain and body. You will learn how it triggers the release of hormones that govern your energy, mood, and stress resilience. You will understand its power to act as a prescription-free antidepressant, a potent focus aid, and the most important ingredient for a night of deep, restorative sleep. Research shows that just one hour of outdoor light in the morning can reduce depression symptoms by 50% compared to staying indoors.

Then, I will give you the protocol. It is a simple, clear, and actionable set of instructions for getting your daily dose of morning light, no matter where you live or how busy you are. This is a clinical prescription right under our feet, or rather, just over our heads.

This is your first, most important step in taking back your biology from the clutches of an indoor world that is systematically depleting it. Think of this as your morning reset. Don't let your 7% slip past unnoticed.

The Why: Setting Your Master Clock for Energy and Focus

The primary mechanism being disrupted by our indoor lives is the most ancient and fundamental rhythm of all life on Earth: the circadian rhythm (see Glossary).

Outdoor Rx does not depend on gadgets or apps. Your body already carries the most advanced timing system on Earth. It is your circadian rhythm.

This internal clock sets the pace for everything from energy to digestion. In adults, it runs a little longer than a full day (24.2 hours), so it needs a fresh reset every morning. That reset process is called entrainment, and it works best when it syncs with natural light.

Modern life can knock this system far off course. Screens at night, indoor lighting, and constant rushing confuse the signals your body depends on. When your rhythm drifts, so does everything else. Sleep becomes shallow. Hormones wobble. Metabolism slows. Even your immune system falls out of step.

Your circadian rhythm decides when you feel awake, when you feel hungry, and when your body shifts into repair mode. When you bring it back into alignment, you feel the difference fast.

The Indoor Epidemic has systematically corrupted this operating system. By depriving ourselves of bright, natural daylight and flooding our nights with stimulating content and bright blue light from screens and bulbs, we have sent our internal clocks into a state of chronic, disorienting jet lag. Blue light after dark can suppress our natural sleep hormone, melatonin, by up to 80%, delaying the onset of sleep and contributing to many downstream problems.

> **Watercooler Fact:**
>
> **The Longevity Dosage: You need at least 120 minutes outdoors weekly to see any health gains: aim for 300 minutes to hit optimal survival and healthspan.**

The result is the fatigue, brain fog, and low-grade depression that have become the background noise of modern life. Your mission begins with restoring the integrity of this system. And your primary weapon is light.

My patient Sarah's life had narrowed to a microscopic view of neural circuits and grant applications. Brilliant yet perpetually wired, she felt tired and wired, burning the late-night laptop blue light. Her circadian rhythms were gone, without sunrise or natural light exposure, which fragmented her focus and made her feel inadequate and incompetent.

But she turned it around. She made herself get out the door to a nearby park for 15 minutes before powering on her computer. She took her phone for safety, but she tried to make it just her and the dawn. That simple change started an antidepressant cascade: her cortisol (see Glossary) dropped, anxiety went down, and her working memory actually improved.

Cutting off her own work at night with a hard stop three hours before bed allowed her melatonin to kick in like clockwork, getting her back on the road to deep sleep. Over weeks, the self-doubt seemed to subside: she powered through experiments with a resilience she thought she'd lost.

> **Watercooler Fact:**
> Blue Light Sleep Delay: Evening blue light exposure can delay melatonin release by 1.5 hours, fragmenting sleep and leaving you less rested.

The SCN: Your Brain's Master Clock: The CEO of Time

Deep within your brain, nestled in a region of the hypothalamus, and smaller than a grain of rice, lies a tiny yet measurably powerful cluster of approximately 20,000 nerve cells. That is your body's CEO of time: the suprachiasmatic nucleus (SCN) (see Glossary) or Master Clock (see Glossary). It syncs every organ and hormone to the sun. When it's off, your whole system falls out of step.

When this command tower receives a strong, consistent signal, the system runs smoothly. Hormones are released at the right times. Your energy peaks and dips in rhythm with the day. Metabolism, immune function, and even cellular repair are timed for maximum efficiency. You feel aligned, focused, and resilient.

But the tower's guidance is scrambled when light cues are erratic or absent, as they often are indoors. Your internal systems fall out of sync. It's like a city running on a broken grid: power surges here, brownouts there.

The result is biological confusion, sluggish metabolism, disrupted sleep, and poor mental focus. The Master Clock's most reliable calibration tool? Morning light entering your eyes. It's the reset button your entire body depends on.

> **Watercooler Fact:**
>
> Morning Light Reset: Light is a nutrient. Just 15 minutes of real morning sunlight provides more light information to your brain than an entire day under office fluorescents.

The Light Signal: A High-Priority Biological Command

The light that matters for this purpose is not just any light. The way your brain detects it has nothing to do with forming images. A third class of photoreceptor cells, discovered only recently, does this work. They are called intrinsically photosensitive retinal ganglion cells (ipRGCs) (see Glossary) or your light-sensing cells.

Light-sensing cells are separate from the rods and cones you use for vision. Their job is to act as a light meter for the brain and, unlike rods and cones, they are central to your body's circadian rhythm. Light-sensing cells report the overall brightness and color of the light around you directly to the Master Clock that governs your circadian rhythm.

These light-sensing cells are uniquely sensitive to the specific wavelengths of blue and green light that fill the sky in the hours after sunrise. This early brightness signal tells your brain that the day has begun. It sets the timing for your hormones, metabolism, and energy for the next 24 hours.

This is an important point. The warm, orange glow of a sunrise is beautiful, but the magical biological signal your brain is waiting for happens as the sun gets higher in the sky and bathes the atmosphere in this blue-rich light. That's true even on a heavily overcast day. The intensity and spectral quality of outdoor light on a gloomy, gray morning is still many times more powerful and biologically effective than the light from any standard indoor bulb.

When this specific quality of light hits the light-sensing cells in your eyes, it triggers an electrochemical signal. That signal travels along a dedicated neural pathway, the retinohypothalamic tract directly to the Master Clock. This isn't a polite nudge from your brain: it's a big wake-up call, literally. Your body undergoes a hard reset, snapping you back into sync with the planet's rhythm. Your biology is shouting, "Day one--let's go!"

The Cortisol Awakening Response (CAR): Igniting Your Daily Engine

One of the first and most critical parts of this wake-up sequence is the Cortisol Awakening Response, or CAR. After receiving the morning light signal, your Master Clock instructs your adrenal glands to release a healthy, strong surge of the hormone cortisol.

Now, cortisol has gotten a bad rap. We usually associate it with chronic stress, and chronically elevated cortisol is damaging. But the morning cortisol pulse is different. It is not the hormone of stress; it is the hormone of action. It is your natural, clean-burning rocket fuel for the day.

This essential cortisol pulse, which should rise by about 50% and peak 30-45 minutes after you wake, is what gets you out of bed feeling alert and ready to engage with the world. It mobilizes glucose for immediate energy. It sharpens your focus. It tunes up your immune system for daytime threats. It helps regulate inflammation (see Glossary). A strong, healthy CAR is a clinical marker of a resilient stress-response system. It's what gives you that feeling of handling whatever the day throws at you.

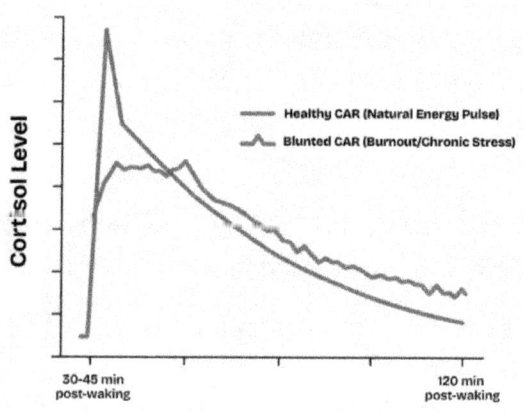

A weak or blunted CAR is one of the most reliable biomarkers of burnout, HPA axis trouble, and depression. It is also the biology behind that crushing morning grogginess and the fog that makes your first thoughts feel slow. This is why so many people reach for a pot of coffee just to feel like themselves again.

If you wake up feeling behind before the day has even started, your morning light signal is failing you. Your brain is not getting the cue it needs to switch fully on. Without that signal, the body cannot mount a strong CAR, and your entire morning feels like a fight. The fix begins the moment you step outside.

Here is the critical, actionable truth: typical indoor lighting, which usually measures a dim 300-500 lux, is not intense enough to trigger this important hormonal cascade. To get the powerful signal, your brain requires, you must expose your eyes to the potent light of the outdoors, which can range from 1,000 lux on an overcast day to over 100,000 lux in direct sun. You cannot hack this with a standard or even most natural light lamps or bulbs. You must go outside. This is your 7% moment.

> **Watercooler Fact:**
> Light Intensity Gap: Your typical office has 300-500 lux of light. Step outside on a cloudy day? You get 1000-2500 lux, up to 5x more.

The Dopamine Connection: Reclaiming Your Focus and Drive

That strong morning pulse of cortisol doesn't just wake you up. It sets in motion an important neurochemical cascade that directly impacts your ability to focus and meet your goals. Specifically, it is foundational for healthy baseline levels of the neuromodulator dopamine.

Dopamine is not just the pleasure molecule. Its real power is drive. It fuels your motivation and your ability to focus. It powers problem-solving. It runs your working memory.

Working memory is your mental workbench. It is not long-term storage. It is the small space in your mind where you hold a phone number, a short list of instructions, or the key points from a meeting. It is the space you use to shape those pieces into a short-term goal. When this system works well, your brain feels sharp and steady.

People with a strong working memory have higher dopamine availability in the prefrontal cortex. This is the part of the brain that runs planning, judgment, and attention. When dopamine is low, working memory drops. You lose your grip on thoughts. You start a task and then forget what you were doing. Even simple projects feel complicated.

This is what the modern world calls distraction. In truth, it is something deeper. Your attention is not broken. It is underfed. Your brain is asking for nourishment, not noise, and the Indoor Epidemic is starving it of the focus it was built to hold.

James was the archetype of digital overload: six glare-filled monitors, a default clenched jaw, and a constant tension headache. He knew his world had gotten smaller, as if he had crippling arthritis, but what crippled him was scrolling and news alerts. Without natural light exposure, his circadian rhythm was disrupted.

His first prescription seemed simple enough: every morning, within 15 minutes of waking, I asked James to step onto his foggy apartment balcony for 15 minutes of even indirect sunlight through the clouds, to reset. Within three days, he felt more energetic (that was his CAR), and his headache improved without all the acetaminophen. His mood improved, and by the fifth day, he slept well for the first time in months, he said.

His second prescription was unexpected too: a 10-minute, phone-free walk in a nearby park to restore focus and give his brain a rest. He dimmed his screen brightness and enabled blue-light filters after 6 p.m. to help his evening wind-down and avoid disrupting it. He was surprised that his trading performance even improved, reflecting the newfound harmony between his biology and his workday.

By ensuring you receive a powerful morning light signal to trigger a healthy CAR, you provide the foundational input your brain needs to synthesize and deploy the dopamine it requires for a day of focused, effective work. This single, simple habit is more potent than any nootropic supplement for enhancing your baseline cognitive performance.

The Serotonin & Mood Link: A Prescription-Free Antidepressant

The benefits of morning light extend deep into your emotional world. The same light signal that triggers cortisol and sets the stage for dopamine also stimulates the production of the neurotransmitter serotonin.

Serotonin is often called the happiness molecule, but its role is more nuanced. It is a powerful regulator of mood, promoting feelings of well-being, calm, and confidence. It helps to manage anxiety and rumination-that pattern of getting stuck in negative thought loops.

The Light Signal Pathway to the Brain

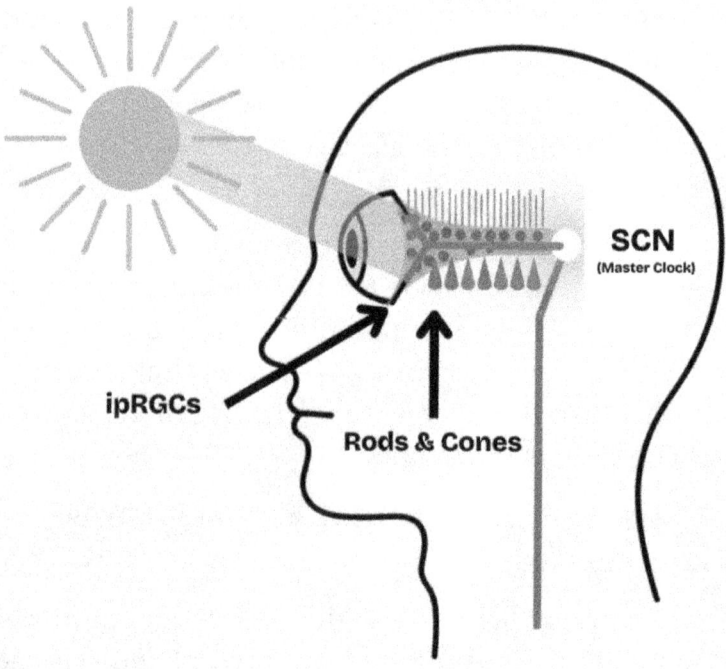

Adequately bright light has real clinical power. In people with nonseasonal major depressive disorder, bright light therapy has performed as well as fluoxetine (Prozac), one of the most prescribed antidepressants in the world. That finding surprised even researchers. It shows how strongly the brain responds to the right kind of light at the right time.

This is not a replacement for medical care when someone is experiencing depression. But it is proof of a larger truth. Light is one of the most potent signals your brain receives each day.

It shapes mood chemistry. It steadies emotional rhythms. And it gives the nervous system the push it needs to lift you out of the low states that the Indoor Epidemic makes so common.

When you deliberately expose yourself to morning sunlight, you are administering a gentle, daily dose of a natural antidepressant.

Setting the Clock for Sleep: The Melatonin Countdown

Finally, and perhaps most counterintuitively, the most important thing you can do to ensure a night of deep, restorative sleep happens the moment you wake up. Getting that powerful blast of morning light is what sets your body's clock for a healthy sleep cycle that night.

The Master Clock uses the morning light signal as its primary anchor to start a countdown timer. Based on this definitive day has begun message, it precisely schedules the release of your primary sleep hormone, melatonin, for 12 to 14 hours later.

It is this carefully timed rise in melatonin in the evening that makes you feel naturally drowsy and physiologically prepared for sleep. It's what allows you to fall asleep easily and transition into the deep, slow-wave sleep stages where your brain and body perform most of their critical repair and detoxification work. A chronic single percent drop in deep sleep stages after age 60 can increase Alzheimer's risk by 27%, highlighting how critical this process is for brain health.

Without a strong, clear morning light anchor, the melatonin signal from the Master Clock becomes weak, muddled, or delayed. This is a primary cause of difficulty falling asleep. You lie in bed, tired but wired, your brain refusing to shut down.

This is your body telling you it never got a clear start signal, so it doesn't know when to start the stop sequence.

The Master Switch for a Longer Life

For years, we've been trained to ask the wrong question about sleep: "How many hours did you get?" While duration does matter, the science now shows it's not the most powerful factor for long-term health. The better question is: "How consistent are your sleep and wake times?"

A landmark study of over 60,000 adults followed for nearly 8 years found that sleep regularity was a stronger predictor of mortality than total hours slept. People who kept the most regular sleep schedules had a dramatically lower risk of death from all causes, including heart disease and cancer, even when their total sleep time wasn't ideal. Consistency beats quantity when it comes to protecting your healthspan. Regular bed and wake times drive resilience and survival in ways hours alone cannot.

Watercooler Fact:

Sleep Consistency: People with regular sleep schedules have a 34% lower risk of heart disease and a 19% lower risk of overall mortality.

Nature exposure works the same way. The line is sharp. Below 120 minutes a week, the body shows no measurable benefit. None. Once you cross that line, the improvements jump. People report a 59 percent higher chance of feeling in good health and a 23 percent boost in well-being.

The curve climbs until it peaks between 200 and 300 minutes per week. That is the longevity plateau: 300 minutes is optimal. That is the full dose for longevity. More time outdoors holds the gains steady but does not push them higher. Five hours a week appears to be the complete prescription.

Americans already average nearly 12 hours a week outdoors. That is almost four times what is required to hit the plateau. But most of those hours are biologically thin. We spend them in parking lots, on sidewalks, in commutes. The problem is not a lack of time. It is a lack of quality.

The difference is in intention. A dog walk in a leafy park, a breakfast on the patio under the morning sky, a lunch break under trees: these minutes carry weight. They count toward the clinical minimum of 120 and build toward the best zone of 200 to 300 minutes. The body recognizes them and responds.

The numbers are clear enough to shape health policy worldwide. In Canada, doctors prescribe official park passes. In Scotland, family doctors issue nature prescriptions as part of standard care. In Japan, Shinrin-yoku (forest bathing) is endorsed by the Ministry of Health. Korea and Singapore have built forest therapy into their national health systems. The World Health Organization now lists 120 minutes a week in nature as a global public health guideline, alongside exercise and nutrition.

The message is not to create more time. It is to repurpose the time you already have. Americans are already outdoors far longer than they realize. The task is to claim two of those hours intentionally, then push toward five. That is all it takes to capture the full survival benefit.

> **Watercooler Fact:**
> Vitamin D Window: Morning light primes your skin's Vitamin D receptors; midday UVB rays flip the biochemical switch to actually produce it.

This discovery is the backbone of the Outdoor Rx system, and it begins first thing in the morning. Morning sunlight is the most powerful signal you can send to your body's Master Clock. It's not just a gentle wake-up. It's a critical biological command that locks in your 24-hour rhythm with solar precision. Once that signal is delivered, every cell in your body marches in time: hormones, metabolism, mood, attention, and recovery.

By anchoring your wake time with morning light, you're flipping the master switch that protects your long-term health. The other anchor, which is honoring dusk and protecting darkness, completes the cycle, and we'll return to it in Chapter 7. But know this: the most important step you can take for your longevity and vitality happens at the start of your day.

The How-To (Your Mission): The Morning Light Protocol

The protocol is simple, but every detail matters. Your mission is to get direct, unfiltered outdoor daylight into your eyes within 60-90 minutes of waking, every single day. Consistency is your greatest ally.

Mission Checklist: A Step-by-Step Guide

Step 1: The Urgency of Timing

Your window of opportunity is the first 60 to 90 minutes after waking. The sooner you can get outside, the stronger the signal will be. Don't delay. This isn't something to fit in later when you have time. The biological window opens after waking and begins to close quickly. Think of it like a train leaving the station; you need to be on it.

Step 2: Defeating the Digital Inertia

The greatest enemy of this mission is your smartphone. The ingrained habit of rolling over, grabbing your phone, and scrolling through emails, news, or social media is a powerful form of inertia. It floods your brain with cortisol for all the wrong reasons and keeps you indoors during the most critical biological window of the day.

You need to notice the pattern and make a conscious choice to shift it.

Use an analog alarm clock to avoid screen creep, and keep your Outdoor Rx journal by your bed to catch your thoughts before your phone does. Make a pact with yourself: my biology comes first. The screen can wait 10 minutes; your circadian rhythm cannot. Look outside before you look at a screen in the morning.

Step 3: Location, Location, Location (The Urban Dweller's Edition)

"Get outside" can sound daunting if you live on the 20th floor of an apartment building. But remember, the mission is to see the sky.

For the Apartment Dweller: Your mission is to get to a place where you can see a large patch of open sky. This could be a balcony, a rooftop (if accessible and safe), or simply walking out the front door of your building and standing on the sidewalk. If you're in an urban canyon surrounded by tall buildings, walk to the nearest street corner or small pocket park where the view opens up.

For the Suburbanite: You have an advantage. Step out onto your porch, your deck, or into your backyard. A few minutes in your bathrobe with a cup of coffee or tea is all it takes.

The Key Principle: You are aiming for photons from the sky to enter your eyes. You don't need to be in a pristine forest. The light in a city park is just as biologically effective as the light on a mountaintop.

Steps 4 & 5: The No-Filter Rule (Sunglasses and Windows)

For this mission to succeed, the specific wavelengths of light must reach your retinas unimpeded. This means two things:

No Sunglasses: Sunglasses are designed to block light, and they work! Wearing them during this critical window is like trying to send an important email to your brain with the Wi-Fi off. Take them off: if you rely on tinted prescription glasses, switch to clear lenses for your morning session, or use contacts. Let nothing stand between your eyes and the sky. But don't look directly at the sun!

No Windows: Do not try to do this through a window, even a bright, sunny one. Glass filters out much of the UVA and UVB wavelengths that contribute to the light's power. You must be physically outdoors, with no glass between you and the sky.

Your prescription eyeglasses or contact lenses are perfectly fine.

Doctor It Up: You might worry that UV-blocking contact lenses interfere with your circadian rhythm's response to morning light. This concern is misplaced. Your Master Clock is set by specialized retinal cells maximally sensitive to blue-green light around 480 nm, not UV light. UV-blocking contacts filter harmful UV radiation while allowing vital blue-green wavelengths through unimpeded. Wearing standard UV-blocking contacts without sunglasses in the morning maximizes both safety and circadian entrainment.

Asking for non-UV-blocking lenses would be medically inadvisable. Chronic UV exposure is strongly linked to cataracts, photokeratitis, and Age-Related Macular Degeneration (AMD), a leading cause of blindness. Clinical data show that UV-blocking contact lens wearers have significantly greater macular pigment density, a key defense against AMD (0.41 vs. 0.33, $p < 0.05$). Ask your optometrist to confirm your lenses transmit 480 nm light and prescribe the highest certified UV protection available, ideally FDA Class 1, to protect your vision long term.

Step 6: Dosing Your Light Correctly

The duration you need depends on the intensity of the light, which varies with weather, time of year, and your latitude.

Bright, Clear Sunny Day: On a day with clear blue skies, you only need 10-15 minutes.

Partly Cloudy or Hazy: When there's a bit of cloud cover, you need to extend your exposure to compensate. Aim for 15-20 minutes.

Very Overcast, Grey, or Light Rain: It may seem counterintuitive, but you need the most exposure on the darkest days. These days, you need 20-30 minutes, or even longer. Find a covered porch, a bus stop shelter, or use an umbrella.

Step 7: The Sensory Micro-Dose

To amplify the benefits of this protocol, don't just stand there passively. Use these few minutes to engage your senses. This practice helps to down-regulate your nervous system and pull you out of the anxious, ruminating thoughts that often plague our mornings. I recommend a simple, one-minute meditation for each sense:

Listen (1 Minute): Close your eyes. First, notice the sound closest to you, perhaps the sound of your own breathing. Then expand your awareness of sounds farther away. Can you isolate the song of a specific bird? The rustle of leaves? The distant hum of traffic? Try to identify three sounds.

See (1 Minute): Let your gaze rest on a single natural object without staring. Notice the detailed pattern of veins on a single leaf, the texture of a tree's bark, the shape of a passing cloud. Appreciate its complexity.

Feel (1 Minute): Bring your awareness to your skin. Can you feel the air temperature on your cheeks? A gentle breeze on your arms? Sun warmth on your neck? Notice the sensation of your feet on the ground.

Smell (1 Minute): Take a conscious breath in through your nose. What does the morning smell like? Can you smell damp earth, blooming flowers, or the clean scent of rain in the air?

Step 8: Finish with Intention

Before you head back inside to the demands of your day, take one final, slow, deep breath. Take just 30 seconds to do a quick internal scan. Do you notice any shift, however small, in your level of alertness, energy, or mood? Acknowledge it. This conscious act of noticing the positive feedback is a form of self-reinforcement that makes the habit much more likely to stick. Log the shift right away in your Outdoor Rx journal or "Morning Vibe Check" to lock in the win and track your momentum against digital fatigue.

Nature Notes & Doctor It Up! Your Advanced Mission Briefing

Once you've mastered the basic protocol, you can begin to layer in more advanced techniques to further enhance your cognitive performance and stress resilience.

Doctor It Up #1: The Morning Power Pair (Light + Cold)

The cortisol and dopamine cascade triggered by morning light is powerful on its own. But if you want to create a state of truly unparalleled focus and mental clarity, pair it with Deliberate Cold Exposure. Submerging your body in cold water causes a massive, sustained increase in dopamine and norepinephrine, the neurochemicals required for alertness, focus, and drive.

The Protocol: Complete your morning light session as described above. Then, 30 to 60 minutes later, take a cold shower or, if you have access, a cold plunge. The duration should be between one and three minutes. The water temperature should be uncomfortable enough that you have to use your willpower to stay in, but not so cold that it is painful or unsafe. For most people, a temperature between 40 and 50°F (4 and 10°C) is effective.

This potent one-two punch, light followed by cold, is one of the most effective natural combinations for priming your brain and body to perform their best.

Doctor It Up #2: The Afternoon Recharge (Non-Sleep Deep Rest --NSDR)

Even with a perfect morning routine, the demands of modern work can leave you with an afternoon slump in energy and focus. The typical response is to reach for more caffeine or sugar.

A far more effective tool is Non-Sleep Deep Rest (NSDR), also known as yoga nidra. It's not a nap: you don't fall asleep. You just lie down, close your eyes, and (typically) listen to a guided script with breathing cues and gentle body scans. NSDR systematically relaxes your body and allows your brain to enter a restorative, sleep-like state, which gives you improved energy and stress levels.

Research has shown that a single ten to 20 minute session of NSDR or yoga nidra can increase baseline dopamine levels in key brain regions by up to 60%. This replenishes your focus capacity and helps you finish your day strong, without interfering with your ability to sleep later that night, as afternoon energy drinks can.

The Protocol: When you feel that 3 p.m. slump hitting, find a quiet place where you can lie down for ten to 20 minutes without being disturbed. Use an app or a free YouTube script to guide you through the process.

Doctor It Up #3: Nutritional Support for Dopamine & Working Memory

While behavioral tools should always be your first line of defense, certain supplements can provide more support for your dopamine system, especially if you know your baseline levels are low.

L-Tyrosine: This amino acid is a direct precursor to dopamine. Supplementing with L-Tyrosine can increase the raw materials your brain has available to produce dopamine, which has been shown in studies to improve working memory. The typical starting dose is 500 mg.

Mucuna Pruriens: This legume, also known as velvet bean, contains L-Dopa, which is the direct molecular precursor to dopamine. This makes it a potent way to increase dopamine levels.

Important Caveat: Approach these supplements with caution and respect. Some people can experience a crash when the effects wear off. Use them infrequently, not nightly, and never when sleep-deprived. Too-high dopamine can backfire, disrupting sleep or triggering irritability. As always, research, test, and use the supplements in therapeutic trials: know your baseline before you start, how long you expect to use them, and when you would stop them if they're not working. Look for interactions using openevidence.com and your clinicians.

Doctor It Up #4: Troubleshooting & Frequently Asked Questions

"What if I wake up hours before the sun?" This is common for shift workers or early risers. The protocol is to turn on as many bright artificial lights as you can indoors when you wake up.

This provides an initial, although weaker, signal to your brain. Then, when the sun is actually up, you must go outside and get your dose of true daylight to properly anchor the rhythm.

"What about my Vitamin D?" Morning light sets your internal biological clock by stimulating receptors in your eyes. But Vitamin D isn't part of that process: it depends on light on your skin. Specifically, UVB rays from the midday sun, when UVB is most available, trigger Vitamin D production. Morning light syncs your circadian rhythm, but it is midday sun that fuels your Vitamin D levels.

"What about the bad air?" A valid concern, especially in cities. However, indoor air quality is often significantly worse than outdoor air. High levels of indoor carbon dioxide (CO_2) can impair cognitive function by up to 50%. Your short morning sun session is also a fresh-air session that helps clear your head, literally by reducing CO_2 buildup. Check your local air quality index if you have concerns. Usually, the benefits of the light far outweigh the risks of a short exposure.

Watercooler Fact:

Indoor Air Quality: The average home has 5x more pollutants than outdoor air, even in cities.

Doctor It Up! #5: The 20-5-3 Advanced Dosing Plan

Neuroscientist Dr. Rachel Hopman coined the 20-5-3 reminder as a repair plan for the modern brain: our biology still expects sunlight, silence, and space. She suggests:

- 20 minutes in nature three times a week to lower cortisol and sharpen focus
- 5 hours each month in wilder places to reset your nervous system
- 3 days fully off-grid each year to restore creativity and quiet the noise.

Nature Note: I live in Southern California, where wildfires make bad air undeniable. But nationwide, the average home has up to five times more pollutants than the air outside. Shoes drag in lead, pesticides, and heavy metals. Mix their dust with flame-retardant chemicals from furniture, phthalates from plastics, and volatile organic compounds from paints and sprays, and you have toxic indoor air. Hormone disruption, airway irritation, and impaired child development are associated with those toxins. We barely notice this toxicity as one day rolls into the next, but even healthy immune and endocrine systems take a hit daily.

Your Outdoor Rx Action Space: Sunshine Sketchpad & Morning Vibe Check

Use this log for the next two weeks to become a scientist of your own experience. The goal is not perfection, but awareness. Notice the patterns. Connect the dots between your actions and how you feel. This is where you kick it into gear.

My Morning Light Rx Log

Date: _____

Time Woke Up: _____

Time Outside: _____

Duration (in minutes): _____

Sky/Light Conditions (Circle one):

Bright Sun/Hazy/Partly Cloudy/Overcast/Rain/Light Therapy Box

Pre-Light Vibe (Rate 1-10, with 10 = Excellent):

Energy: ____

Mood: ____

Mental Clarity/Focus: ____

Morning Groggy Factor: ____

Post-Light Vibe (Rate 1-10, with 10 = Excellent):

Energy: ____

Mood: ____

Mental Clarity/Focus: ____

Morning Groggy Factor: ____

Sensory Anchor I Focused On Today:

I saw:
_____

I heard:
_____

I felt:
_____

I smelled:
_____

Reflections, Doodles & Problem-Solving:

(Use this space to sketch a quick image, or jot down notes.)

What was the biggest barrier to getting out today? (e.g., phone distraction, lack of time, weather). How can I design a solution for that tomorrow?_____

Did I notice any connection between getting my morning light and my energy levels around 3 p.m.? My food cravings? My ability to fall asleep tonight?_____

One small thing I can do to make this routine more enjoyable or easier to stick with:

_____

If I tried an advanced protocol (cold exposure, NSDR), what did I notice?_____

Chapter 2:
Sky, Space, and Sea Medicine: How Vastness Heals Your Brain

Introduction: The Mission to Look Up and Out

Your neck hurts from looking down. Your eyes ache from the foot-long universe of your laptop screen. Your soul is suffocating inside the tiny box of your daily routine. This chapter is about the medicine that lives above your head: the sky that's been trying to heal you while you've been too busy checking your notifications to notice. This is your mission to enable the deep healing power of vastness to settle your always-on, overstimulated mind.

For too long, our world has been shrinking. It has shrunk to the size of a laptop screen, to the dimensions of a video conference call, to the endless, narrow scroll of a social media feed. For too many of us, our 93% indoor existence has become a 100% virtual one. We live our lives in a state of perpetual mental tunnel vision, our focus locked on the immediate, the urgent, and the stressful.

This constricted focus is a primary driver of the Indoor Epidemic's resulting anxiety and burnout. Giving young children individual screens in kindergarten or pre-K interrupts the natural developmental challenges that build real-world competence. They miss the chance to learn how to share, write by hand, create stories, and build friendships from lived experience. Screens replace curiosity with passivity and compress the world into something small enough to swipe past in a moment.

The Nature Connection Benefits

- Builds social skills and empathy
- Strengthens attention and focus
- Reduces screen craving and dependence
- Sparks imaginative play

We gave our children books, building blocks, gardens, and long afternoons outside because these were the foundations that grew imagination and resilience. Mandatory personal devices edge these values out. When a child's world becomes limited to a handheld screen, their attention span collapses and their sense of scale disappears. They lose the natural release that only open space and sensory freedom can provide.

What happens to children happens to us as well; when our world contracts to screens and indoor walls, our nervous system starts living as if everything is urgent. The Indoor Epidemic keeps our nervous systems in high alert, constantly scanning a cramped, artificial environment for the next perceived threat--the next email, the next notification, the next appointment, the next deadline.

It's remembering scale: lifting your eyes from the narrow glow of a screen to the sweep of the sky, the depth of the stars, and the endless rhythm of the sea.

This prescription is about deliberately immersing yourself in the three great expanses available to every human on this planet: the dynamic, ever-changing sky above you; the infinite, humbling depth of night space; and the rhythmic power of the sea and its freshwater counterparts.

Whether it's the quiet, soul-stirring wonder of a starry sky, the meditative lull of waves lapping the shore, or the sheer immensity of a sunrise sky turning from pale lavender to liquid fire, engaging with these vast natural canvases offers deep psychological and physiological relief.

There's no need to travel to exotic beaches or remote, light-pollution-free mountaintops. The power of this prescription lies in its accessibility. To capture these awe-inspiring moments with focused intention, use an actual film camera or quick-snap camera: it encourages you to slow down and thoughtfully compose each shot. You can begin this mission right where you are--on your porch, in your backyard, from a bench in a city park, or by the edge of a local river or pond.

When we engage with the vastness of sky, space, or sea, we activate ancient neural circuits designed to register scale and trigger awe. Awe is not a luxury; it is a biologically potent state. It lowers stress reactivity, regulates the autonomic nervous system, and reduces self-focus. Awe is powerful: it triggers compassion, gratitude, and admiration.

Light itself is one of awe's most consistent triggers. At dawn and dusk, our boundary moments of the day, changing light floods the brain's reward circuits, syncing us with the planet's own circadian rhythms and evoking awe as reliably as any pharmacologic signal.

These effects matter for healthspan. Feelings of isolation, fear, and anxiety accelerate cognitive decline and physical disease, but awe reliably counteracts them. Even simple practices, such as awe walks described in Forest-Bathing studies, increase positive affect, enhance social connection, and improve markers linked to longevity. Awe is a measurable input for resilience and longer life.

Light Optimization Protocol

- Get 10 minutes of morning light before 10 a.m.
- Reduce glare from overhead LEDs
- Use warm, indirect light in the evenings
- Dim lights two hours before bed

The Why: The Neurological Case for Looking Up and Out

The modern indoor world is a cage for your perception. Your attention and consciousness are relentlessly drawn inward and downward, and funneled into the tight, glowing confines of a screen. Your auditory world is a cacophony of digital pings and urban noise. Your sense of self, under the constant pressure of productivity and social comparison, has become a looped recording of worries, to-do lists, and self-criticism.

The modern struggle, however, often manifests as mental tunnel vision, caused by constant information bombardment and digital overwhelm. Nature can actively restore and prevent this.

This is the state of mental tunnel vision, a core pathology of the Indoor Epidemic. This state physically and neurologically fosters anxiety, burnout, and a deep sense of disconnection.

To break free, we need a clear shift in how we direct our attention. We have to guide it intentionally upward and outward so the world can open back up again. And for some of us, chronically inside, so we can open back up to the world.

The practices in this chapter (greeting the sky, making space for space, seeking the sea) may sound simple and even poetic. But make no mistake: they are potent, evidence-based neurological interventions. What ancient sailors, desert wanderers, and stargazers have always known in their bones, modern neuroscience is now beginning to map.

Engaging with the vastness of the sky, space, and sea triggers a cascade of powerful, beneficial changes in your brain and body. Those changes dial down ego noise, regulate your nervous system, repair visual strain, and restore a sense of perspective required for true well-being. This is not soft wellness; this is hard science.

As you already know, prolonged indoor living has measurable cognitive and physiological costs. These five evidence-based Outdoor Rx practices drawn directly from clinical science can help:

1. Awe and the Quieting of the Self: Your Brain on Vastness

First, I've already mentioned awe, but it deserves more detail. Awe is the feeling that washes over you in the presence of something vast, something that transcends your ordinary frame of reference and forces you to update your mental model of what is possible. It is the feeling of looking up at a sky impossibly dense with stars, of standing at the edge of the Grand Canyon, or of watching a massive thunderhead build on the horizon. It is the emotion that makes you feel, in the best way, small.

This small-self experience is not only psychological. Awe slows the heart, deepens the breath, and produces a calm shift in the body. These are classic signs of vagus nerve activation. When the vagus nerve fires, it signals safety and helps quiet the overactive Default Mode Network (DMN) or the Narrator of me. The vagus redirects attention away from self-focused chatter to the vast sensory world around you. This reset builds calmness, connection, and compassion, benefiting both your physiology and emotions. See Glossary for vagus nerve, awe and DMN explanations.

> **Watercooler Fact:**
> Awe's Anti-Inflammatory Power: Experiences of awe, like watching a sunset reduce inflammatory markers and strengthen immune resilience.

The Default Mode Network: Your Brain's Storyteller

When your mind wanders while daydreaming, replaying the past, or worrying about the future, that's your Narrator of me. For too many of my patients, it's not a quiet background hum; it's a full-blown, self-obsessed show on Broadway running 24/7, fueling anxiety and rumination. The Narrator is the seat of your ego. It is the narrator of your life, the part of you that constantly constructs and maintains the story of me: my worries, my goals, my regrets, my identity.

In a healthy, balanced brain, the Narrator is a useful tool. It allows for self-reflection, planning, and creativity. But in our modern world, for many people, the Narrator has become overactive and dysfunctional. It has become a relentless engine of rumination: that toxic mental habit of getting stuck in repetitive, negative, self-referential thought loops. It is the voice in your head that replays an awkward conversation on a loop, that obsesses over a future worry, or that criticizes your past mistakes. An overactive Narrator is a hallmark of anxiety, depression, and the constant underlying feeling of being stuck that so many of my patients experience.

Neurological Pattern Interrupt

This is where the power of vastness comes in. Experiences of awe act as a powerful pattern interrupt for the overactive Narrator. When your brain is confronted with the immense scale of the ocean or the night sky, it is forced to shift its resources away from the internal chatter of the self and toward the processing of the overwhelming new sensory information.

Research has shown this directly. Neuroimaging studies have found that inducing states of awe in participants leads to a significant and immediate decrease in Narrator activity. And the Narrator of me, me, me is momentarily silenced. In that quiet space, something remarkable happens. Participants in these studies report feeling less focused on their individual problems, more connected to the world around them, and more generous toward others. The shrinking of the self opens up space for a connection to something larger.

This quieting of the Narrator of me is not just a fleeting feeling. It seems to have lasting benefits. By regularly engaging in practices that induce awe like the ones in this chapter you are training your brain to be less self-obsessed and more present. You are weakening the neural pathways of rumination and strengthening the pathways of connection and wonder. You are getting out of your own head.

Patient Case: Michael, the Accountant Trapped in a Spreadsheet

Let me tell you about Michael. At 42, Michael was a successful tax accountant. His entire professional life was lived within the tight, logical, and demanding limits of a spreadsheet. His focus was narrow, detailed, and inward-looking. He came complaining of chronic anxiety, a persistent feeling of pressure in his chest, and what he described as mental tunnel vision.

"It's like I'm stuck inside my screen," he told me. "Even when I'm not working, my brain is just crunching numbers, replaying meetings, stressing over emails. I can't shut it off. It's like my own thoughts are attacking me."

Michael was suffering from a pathologically overactive Default Mode Network (DMN). His brain's narrator had become a tyrannical accountant, constantly auditing his life for errors and potential disasters. The first prescription I gave him had nothing to do with medication or therapy. It was a mission: "For the next two weeks, I want you to leave your office at lunch, drive 10 minutes to the bluffs overlooking the ocean, and just sit in your car and look at the water for 15 minutes. No phone, no podcast, no agenda."

At first, he was resistant. It felt unproductive, a waste of billable hours. But after a few days, he reported a change. "It's the weirdest thing," he said. "For the first five minutes, my brain is buzzing. But then... it's like the ocean just... erases the spreadsheet. My problems don't disappear, but they seem less important. The knot in my chest seems to drop away."

What Michael was describing was the direct, felt experience of awe deactivating his Narrator of me. The vastness of the Pacific

Ocean was providing a more compelling signal than the internal chatter of his own anxiety. He was, for the first time in years, getting a break from himself.

2. The Science of Blue Mind: Your Brain on Water

For centuries, poets, artists, and philosophers have been drawn to water, sensing its significant ability to soothe the soul and inspire the mind. Now, modern science is understanding why. Marine biologist Dr. Wallace J. Nichols brilliantly synthesized this emerging field of research, coining the term Blue Mind (see Glossary) to describe the "mildly meditative state characterized by calm, peace, unity, and a sense of general happiness and satisfaction with life in the moment" that is triggered by proximity to water.

This is not just a pleasant emotional state. It is a complex and powerful neurochemical and electrical shift in the brain. Being near, in, on, or under water seems to be a direct trigger for a cascade of positive neurological events.

> **Watercooler Fact:**
>
> Blue Mind Effect: Being near water triggers a mildly meditative state that measurably lowers blood pressure and heart rate.

Let me tell you about Maya, a thirty-something corporate strategist from Chicago who never considered herself the outdoorsy type. But after a miscarriage left her numb and sleepless, she started walking the perimeter of Lake Michigan near downtown every morning before work. Some days, she stormed along the shoreline in rage. Other days, the waves did the weeping for her. She didn't call it therapy. She just knew that when she was near the water, she could breathe again.

This isn't just poetry. It's measurable biology. In recent research from Vienna, participants lay in fMRI scanners while receiving mild electric shocks. When they watched virtual lake scenes instead of city streets, the brain regions that process pain signals became markedly less active. Nature didn't just distract them. It changed how their brains registered pain in real time.

The Neurochemistry of Calm and Connection

When we are in a state of Blue Mind, our brain chemistry literally shifts. The sight, sound, and touch of water activate the parasympathetic nervous system, dampen the hypothalamic stress circuits, and rebalance neural pathways toward safety, reward, and connection.

Cortisol (see Glossary) Drops: Just as we saw with Forest Bathing, being in or near water has been shown to lower levels of the stress hormone cortisol. The gentle, rhythmic sensory inputs of water (the sound, sight, and feeling of it on our skin) signal safety to our nervous system, allowing it to downregulate the stress response.

Dopamine (see Glossary) and Serotonin Rise: Proximity to water helps create feelings of pleasure and positive anticipation, prompting the brain to release dopamine. Simultaneously, the tranquil and rejuvenating qualities of blue spaces boost serotonin levels, the neurotransmitter responsible for promoting well-being and satisfaction. Your brain recognizes a pleasant environment, and your brain responds with the right neurotransmitters.

Oxytocin (see Glossary), the Bonding Hormone, Flows: Water also increases levels of oxytocin. This is the hormone responsible for feelings of trust, empathy, and social connection. It's what makes us feel bonded to our loved ones. This explains why shared experiences by the water-a family beach trip, a conversation with a friend by a river-often feel so deeply connective and memorable.

The Brainwave Shift: Entering a Meditative State

Beyond just chemistry, being near water also changes the electrical activity of your brain. Using EEG technology, researchers can observe that proximity to water usually shifts our brainwaves from the high-frequency, agitated state of beta waves (associated with active, focused thought and anxiety) to the slower, more coherent state of alpha and theta waves.

Alpha waves are the signature of a brain that is awake but deeply relaxed and inwardly focused, a state often achieved during meditation. Theta waves are associated with creativity, intuition, and the twilight state between waking and sleeping. This is why a walk on the beach feels so meditative, and why our best ideas often seem to surface while we stare out at the ocean. Our brain is literally entering a different, more receptive state of consciousness. It is moving from the frantic Red Mind of our stressed, overstimulated daily lives to the calm, clear, creative state of Blue Mind.

Think of Red Mind as your brain's danger radar stuck on high alert by the endless pings, deadlines, and demands of your device and modern life. It's a sort of Code Red that lives in the background of your brain: the constant jitter of fight-or-flight mode that fractures attention and floods you with stress hormones. By deliberately shifting into Blue Mind through simple practices like the Sky Diary, you give your Red Mind a much-needed timeout, restoring balance and allowing genuine rest and repair to take hold.

This effect is so powerful that it can be triggered even by virtual or auditory exposure to water. Studies have shown that simply listening to high-quality recordings of ocean waves or gentle rain can reduce sympathetic nervous system activity and lower heart rate. For urban dwellers with limited access to natural water bodies, a high-quality nature-sound app featuring the sound of the sea becomes an important tool in the arsenal against stress.

3. The Horizon as Eye Medicine: Curing Your Screen-Strained Vision

Our crusade against the Indoor Epidemic is also a crusade to save eyesight. One of the most insidious and underappreciated casualties of our screen-bound lives is the physical health of our eyes. Your eyes, like the rest of your body, were not designed for the demands of the modern world. They evolved to scan vast, naturally lit landscapes, to shift focus from near to far, to track movement in a complex, three-dimensional world.

The Dopamine-Light Connection

Bright, natural outdoor light is a powerful biological signal for your eye health. Compelling research has shown that time spent outdoors is the most effective protective factor against the development and progression of myopia in children.

The Myopia Epidemic: Protecting Your Eyesight

At least one mechanism is now reasonably well understood. The human eye is not designed to be locked on close-range targets under dim, artificial light for hours on end. This sustained near work, combined with a lack of bright outdoor light, causes the eyeball to physically elongate over time, shifting the focal point and blurring distant vision.

> **Watercooler Fact:**
> Screen Time and Myopia: Children with more than two hours of daily screen time have triple the risk of developing nearsightedness.

The antidote is elegantly simple: enough time outdoors. One landmark school-based study in Taiwan showed that increasing outdoor time during recess significantly reduced the rate of new nearsightedness cases from 17.65% to 8.41% over a single year. Another study showed that getting 2+ hours of outdoor time daily can drop a child's myopia risk by 50%.

> **Watercooler Fact:**
> Myopia Epidemic: 50% of the world's population will be nearsighted by 2050, largely because of a lack of outdoor light exposure in childhood.

This was a critical prescription for my patient, Michael, the accountant. His screen-induced headaches and eye strain resulted directly from his mental tunnel vision, manifesting as physical tunnel vision. His daily horizon medicine-looking out at the vast expanse of the Pacific Ocean-was not just calming his mind; it was providing a desperately needed therapeutic break for his overworked eyes.

4. The Soundscapes of Vastness: Drowning Out the Noise

Our auditory system is another casualty of the Indoor Epidemic. We live in a world of constant, jarring, artificial noise: the hum of the HVAC system, the drone of traffic, incessant digital pings, the blare of a nearby television. This soundscape keeps our nervous system on low-grade alert. It is the sonic equivalent of a diet of processed junk food.

Natural soundscapes, particularly the sounds associated with vast, open spaces, are the antidote. They are the whole-food diet for your auditory system.

The Rhythmic Power of Water and Wind

The sound of ocean waves is one of the most universally soothing sounds on the planet. The reason lies in its pattern. The sound is not random noise; it is a gentle, predictable, rhythmic pattern of sound and silence.

The slow, steady rhythm of the waves crashing and receding mimics the rhythm of a calm, resting breath or a slow heartbeat. This rhythmic input has a direct and powerful effect on your brain, entraining your own internal rhythms and shifting your nervous system toward a state of parasympathetic calm.

The sound of wind moving through trees or across an open plain has a similar effect. It is a form of pink noise, a type of sound with a consistent frequency that helps mask more jarring background noises, leading to improved relaxation and better sleep quality.

The Informational Richness of Birdsong

Listening to birdsong has also been shown to reduce stress and improve cognitive function. From an evolutionary perspective, the sound of happy, non-alarmed birdsong is a powerful signal of safety to our nervous system. It tells our ancient brain that there are no predators nearby and that it is safe to relax. But the sudden silence of birds or the sound of their alarm calls immediately puts us on high alert.

Studies have found that listening to nature sounds, including birdsong and water sounds, helped participants recover faster from a stressful mental task than listening to urban noise. Other research has shown that exposure to birdsong can improve attention scores by 15% and reduce rumination.

When you deliberately expose yourself to these natural soundscapes, you are doing more than just listening to something pleasant. You are providing your brain with a rich diet of auditory information that is evolutionarily congruent with a state of safety and calm. You are drowning out the stressful noise of the modern world with the healing sounds of nature.

5. Visual Healing: The Restorative Power of Fractals and the Color Blue

Finally, we come to the direct visual healing power of the sky and the sea. This involves two fascinating concepts: the calming effect of natural fractal patterns and the intrinsic psychological impact of the color blue.

Fractals: The Art of Nature

The natural world is filled with patterns that show a property called fractal geometry. This means they show similar, repeating patterns at increasingly smaller or larger scales. Think of the branching of a tree, the shape of a coastline on a map, the structure of a snowflake, or, most relevant to this chapter, the complex, ever-changing patterns of clouds in the sky and waves on the surface of the water.

Our visual system, which coevolved with these patterns over millions of years, seems uniquely attuned to them. Research has shown that viewing these natural fractal patterns has a direct and measurable stress-reducing effect on the body. It lowers physiological stress within minutes, likely by engaging our visual cortex in a way that is both effortless and deeply engaging, inducing a state of soft fascination or involuntary attention, described in more detail in Chapter 3.

The Outdoor Office Toolkit

That restorative power stands in stark contrast to our typical indoor environment: one dominated by straight lines and right angles. Indoors provides little of the stimulation our brains evolved to crave. But rather than relocating your office, The Toolkit can offer fractal-rich views in your workspace. Try a window-facing desk positioned to make it easy to look up at clouds and trees. And a break timer to prompt hourly visual pauses. Use an air purifier that gives you better quality air. Open windows when you can. When you feed your visual system this restorative diet during work breaks, you counteract the visual impoverishment of indoor life.

Watercooler Fact:

> **Biophilic Workplace Boost**
> Offices with natural light and plants have employees with lower blood pressure, fewer sick days, and faster cognitive performance.

The Psychology of Blue

Color psychology has long held that blue is associated with feelings of calm, stability, and peace. While some of this is culturally conditioned, there is a deeper evolutionary reason. For our ancestors, a clear blue sky meant a day of good, safe weather. A clear, clean body of blue water meant a source of life-sustaining hydration. In the natural world, the color blue is overwhelmingly a signal of safety and abundance.

When we look at the vast expanse of a blue sky or a blue ocean, it taps into these ancient, hardwired associations. This is a key part of the Blue Mind theory. The color itself contributes to the overall calming, stress-reducing effect of these environments. In comparative studies, blue spaces (such as oceans, rivers, and lakes) have often been found to outperform green spaces (such as forests and parks) in mood enhancement, particularly for people starting from a high baseline of stress.

The practice of looking up and out at the sky, space, and sea is not a passive act of sightseeing. It is a powerful, multi-modal neurological intervention. It leverages the power of awe to quiet your ego, the science of Blue Mind to calm your chemistry, the mechanics of vision to heal your eyes, and the patterns of nature to soothe your entire system. It is the antidote to the mental tunnel vision of our time. It is your prescription for regaining your perspective.

The How-To (Your Mission)

What follows is not a list of suggestions, but five distinct, yet interconnected, missions. This is about learning to see your world differently. Your mission is to open your horizon.

Mission 1: Greet the Sky

The Objective: This is your first and most fundamental mission in this chapter. It is a direct counteroffensive against the tyranny of the screen.

For most of us, the first thing our eyes focus on in the morning is the glowing rectangle of a smartphone. This act immediately constricts our focus, floods our brains with cortisol-inducing information, and sets a tone of digital dependency for the rest of the day. You need to reclaim this sacred morning window. You will make the vast, dynamic, and naturally lit sky your first screen of the day.

The Protocol: A Guided Morning Ritual

Set the Intention: The night before, make a conscious decision to greet the sky the next morning. This small act of pre-commitment makes all the difference. You might even place a note on your phone or your alarm clock that says, "Look Outside."

Wake Up 10 Minutes Earlier: I know this can sound like a big ask, especially if you are already sleep-deprived. But I promise you, these ten minutes of restorative connection will give you back far more energy than 10 extra minutes of restless sleep. This is an investment, not an expense.

Step Outside: As soon as you can after waking-perhaps after a quick trip to the bathroom or while your coffee is brewing-

physically step outside. A porch, a balcony, a front stoop, even just opening your front door and standing on the threshold, will work.

Look Up and Breathe: Tilt your head back and let your gaze drift upward. Take three slow, deep breaths. On the first breath, simply notice your body standing on the earth. On the second, become aware of the air on your skin. On the third, bring your full, gentle attention to the sky itself.

Become a Sky-Watcher: For the next five to 10 minutes, your only job is to observe. Try to notice the specific quality of the light. Is it the pale, pearly gray of a pre-dawn sky? Is it the fiery orange and soft lavender of a sunrise? Is it a crisp, clear, brilliant blue? Is it a uniform, heavy gray of an overcast day? Don't just label it; try to see the nuances. Watch how the light changes, minute by minute, as the sun climbs higher.

Engage in Cloud-Watching: If there are clouds, treat them as a captivating form of natural art. Notice their shape, their texture, their speed. Are they puffy and cotton-like (cumulus)? Are they thin and wispy (cirrus)? Are they a low, moody blanket (stratus)? Let your imagination play. What do they look like? This is a perfect exercise in soft fascination, allowing your attention to be gently held with no effort.

Creative Examples:

The Overachiever's Micro-Dose: For the person who feels they don't have a minute to spare, this can be done while you are waiting for something else to happen. While you wait for the shower to warm up, step onto your balcony. While you wait for the toaster, stand at your open kitchen door. The key is to make it the first intentional act of your day.

> **Watercooler Fact**
>
> **The Green Heart Effect:** Residents in newly greened neighborhoods saw a **20% drop** in inflammation levels (hs-CRP), often more predictive of heart attack than cholesterol.

The Afternoon Reset: If mornings are impossible, try this in the afternoon. Find a patch of grass, lie on your back (if possible), and just watch the clouds drift by for 10 minutes. This may seem daunting: many people balk. But it is a powerful antidote to the brain fog that often sets in after hours of screen time.

Urban Troubleshooting:

Obstructed Views: If you live in a city canyon surrounded by tall buildings, find the biggest patch of sky you can. This might mean walking to a nearby intersection, a bridge, or a pocket park. It might mean going up to the top floor of your apartment building's stairwell and looking out the window (even through glass is better than nothing if it's your only option). The goal is to see as much of the open expanse as possible.

The Sky Diary Tool: Try this: each day, write just one precise phrase describing what you saw in the sky that morning: amber pre-dawn glow, steel-blue sky with wispy cirrus, or pink horizon fading to gold. This simple habit reinforces circadian signaling and sharpens your attention and focus. With it, you strengthen your internal clock: you're also noticing the beauty and dynamism that is always present, even in the heart of a city.

Mission 2: Make Space for Space

The Objective: This mission is a direct intervention against the tyranny of the ego and the endless chatter of the Narrator of me. By deliberately engaging with the immense, humbling vastness of the night sky, you are providing your brain with a powerful dose of awe.

This experience of feeling small in the face of something immense is a neurological reset button. It quiets the self-referential part of your brain, reduces rumination, and dramatically shifts your perspective, making your own problems seem less overwhelming and all-consuming.

The Protocol: A Guided Stargazing Ritual

Choose Your Night: You do not need a perfectly clear, moonless night in the remote wilderness. Choose one night this week, almost whatever the weather, to make space for space.

The Dark Adaptation: Go outside at night, away from the direct glare of streetlights or porch lights. The mission begins with patience. It takes the human eye about 5-10 minutes to begin to adapt to the dark, and up to 30 minutes to adapt. Stand or sit comfortably and simply let your eyes adjust. Resist the urge to look at your phone, as its bright light will instantly ruin your night vision.

Scan the Sky: After a few minutes, let your gaze drift across the sky. Don't search for anything in particular at first. Just take in the expanse. See what stars, planets, or constellations naturally emerge from the darkness. You might be surprised by what is visible even from a light-polluted area.

Learn One New Thing: This is where you can bring a tool to enhance the experience. Look ahead of time at a stargazing app on your phone (like SkyView Lite, Star Walk, or Stellarium) to find out what is visible that night. Instead of using it to map the stars, go outside and see where a specific planet or constellation is located. Recognizing a constellation creates a sense of familiarity and connection.

The Darkness Ritual: Before you go back inside, perform a simple darkness ritual. Take three slow, conscious breaths. With each exhale, feel your jaw unclench, your shoulders drop, and the tension release from your body. Feel the deep quiet and stillness of the night. Acknowledge your own small, precious place in the vastness of the universe.

Creative Examples:

The Insomniac's Ally: One of my patients, (Anna, later described), began a ritual of watching the moon rise through her east-facing window each night before bed. She called it her unplugging ritual. The slow, silent, predictable movement of the moon became a meditative focus that helped to quiet her racing thoughts. Her sleep and her spirit both improved dramatically.

The Family Sky Picnic: A family I worked with was struggling with screen addiction and a lack of quality time together. Their mission was to create a picnic in the Sunday night sky. They would take blankets and sandwiches out to their backyard, leave their phones inside, and just lie on the grass together, watching the stars come out. It became their sacred time, a space for quiet conversation and shared wonder.

Urban Troubleshooting:

Conquering Light Pollution: Stargazing in a city is a challenge, but it is not impossible. The key is to manage your expectations and work with what you have. You will not see the Milky Way from downtown Manhattan. But you can see the Moon, the brightest planets (Venus, Mars, Jupiter, Saturn), and a surprising number of the brightest stars and most recognizable constellations.

Seek Out Relative Darkness: Find the darkest spot you can access. This might be the middle of a large city park, a local cemetery (if it feels safe and respectful), or even the top floor of a parking garage. The goal is to avoid the direct glare of streetlights.

Let Your Eyes Adapt: This is even more important in the city. Give your eyes at least 15 minutes to adjust to the dark before you expect to see much.

Focus on Bright Targets: Use your stargazing app to identify the brightest objects that should be visible from your location. These will be your primary targets.

Plan a Dark Sky Excursion: Once a month or once a season, consider making a short trip to a designated dark sky park or just a more rural area outside your city. The experience of seeing a truly dark sky can be deeply moving and awe-inspiring, leaving you with an experience that will stay with you for weeks.

Mission 3: Seek the Sea (or Water's Substitute)

The Objective: This mission is about tapping into the multi-sensory healing power of water. Being near, in, on, or under water induces the mildly meditative state called Blue Mind, described above. It's a calming, direct antidote to the frantic, overstimulated Red Mind of our modern lives. Your mission is to find your water, whatever and wherever it is, and allow it to wash over your senses.

The Protocol: A Guided Blue Mind Experience

Find Your Water: The ideal is a large, natural body of water: an ocean, a lake, a wide river. But this mission is designed to be accessible to everyone. Your water could also be a small creek or stream, a park pond, or a public fountain in a city plaza.

Be Still and Listen: Find a comfortable spot to sit or stand near the water's edge. Before you do anything else, just listen. Close your eyes. Notice the sound of the water. Is it the rhythmic, crashing roar of ocean waves? The gentle lapping of a lake against the shore? The steady, burbling flow of a creek? The playful splashing of a fountain? The rhythmic sound of water helps put our brains into a state of synchrony, or groove, subconsciously calming our nervous systems.

Practice Water-Gazing: Now, open your eyes. Let your gaze soften and drift over the water's surface. Don't try to focus on any one thing. Just watch the play of light, the movement of the ripples, the patterns of the currents. It holds your attention gently, without dominating it, allowing your mind to enter a more creative, contemplative state.

Make a Sensory Connection: If safe, make a direct physical connection with the water. Dip your fingers or bare toes in it. Notice its temperature, texture, how it moves against your skin. This tactile input deepens the Blue Mind experience, providing a powerful grounding sensation.

Creative Examples:

The Shower as Sanctuary: The common experience of having great ideas in the shower is a perfect example of a daily Blue Mind moment. The warm water, the white noise, the solitude: it all creates a space for our brains to relax and make creative connections. You can make this even more intentional by consciously paying attention to the water's sensory experience on your skin.

The Fountain Meeting: Urban fountains are underutilized sources of creative and private conversation. The sound of the water creates a natural privacy bubble, allowing you to have an intimate conversation with a friend or colleague. Try holding your next important one-on-one meeting by a fountain instead of in a sterile conference room.

Urban Troubleshooting:

When There's No Real Water: For those in truly water-scarce environments, this mission can be adapted.

Auditory Immersion: Use a high-quality nature sound app or a recording of ocean waves or gentle rain. Play this through headphones while walking or sitting outside. Studies have shown that even auditory exposure to water sounds can evoke a physiological relaxation response, lowering heart rate and skin conductance.

Visual Immersion: Watch a high-definition nature documentary about the ocean. While not as powerful as the real thing, visual stimuli can still trigger some of the positive neurological associations. This can be a useful tool on a day when you are sick or otherwise unable to leave your home.

Create a Blue Mind Map: Take out a map of your city or neighborhood and, using a blue highlighter, mark every single accessible water feature, no matter how small: every public fountain, every pond in a park, every creek, every riverfront path. You might be surprised how much blue is hidden in your concrete jungle. This becomes your personal map for finding quick, accessible doses of Blue Mind.

Mission 4: Use the Horizon as Medicine

The Objective: This is a direct, therapeutic intervention for the physical and mental strain of our screen-bound lives. It is a prescription for both your eyes and your mind. The mission is to shift your focus consciously and regularly from the near-field of your immediate tasks and worries to the expansive, distant horizon.

The Protocol: Two Powerful Practices

1. Horizon Scanning: Your 3-Minute Micro-Break

This is your antidote to digital eye strain and its headaches.

The Protocol: Set a timer for three minutes. Step away from your screen. Find a window or a spot outside where you can see the farthest possible point. This could be a distant hill, a faraway building, or just the point where the sky meets the ground.

For these three minutes, your only job is to let your gaze rest on that distant point. You will physically feel the tiny ciliary muscles inside your eyes, which have been clenched to focus on your screen, finally relax. Do not speak. Do not think about anything you need to solve. Just look.

Who It's For: This is a must-do for my patient, Michael, the accountant, and for any other professional who spends hours a day staring at a screen. I advise them to set a recurring timer on their computer to do this at least once an hour. It is powerful form of physical therapy for your eyes.

2. Horizon Breathing: Your Tool for Overwhelm

This is a powerful practice for moments of acute anxiety or overwhelm.

The Protocol: When you feel everyday stress tightening in your chest, find the horizon. Inhale gently; on the exhale, let your gaze move from your feet out to that far line. Pair a longer exhale with the widening view. The combination breaks the tunnel vision of stress and recruits the vagus nerve, slowing heart rate, easing breath, and releasing the body from high alert.

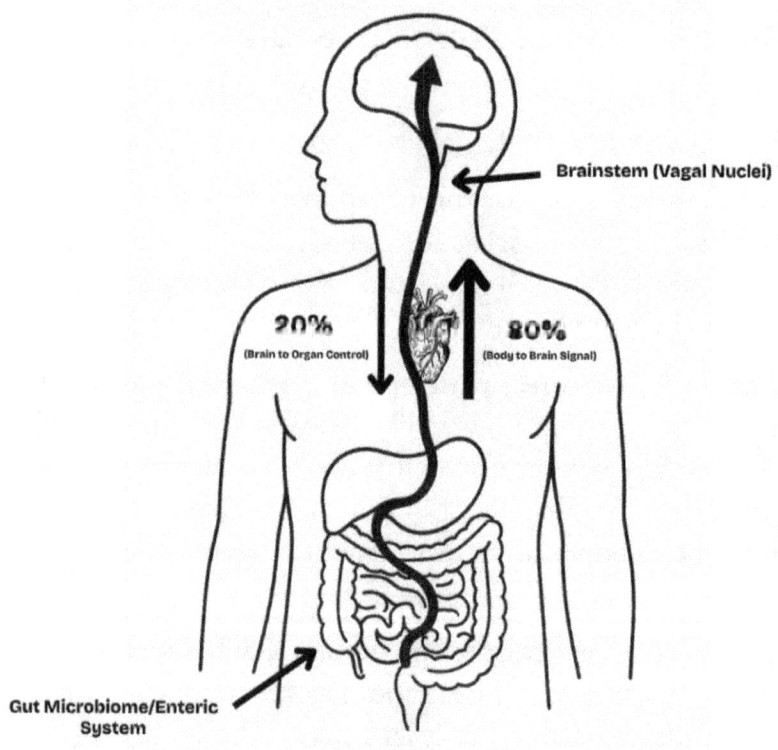

Take a deep breath in, and as you exhale, let your gaze travel slowly from your own feet all the way out to that farthest point. Imagine you are breathing all your stress and worry out toward that distant line. The visual act of expanding your field of view sends a powerful signal to your brain to break out of the tunnel vision of anxiety.

The Boundary: Use the horizon as a psychological boundary. When you look out, imagine placing your immediate problems on your side of the line, with calmness beyond the horizon. This brain's natural tendency is to help you identify stressors, reduce their weight, and restore your perspective. The horizon becomes a visual reminder that what feels overwhelming is limited, while what lies beyond is expansive, stable, and safe.

Urban Troubleshooting:

Finding Your Horizon: This can be a challenge in a city. Your mission is to become a horizon hunter. Where are the places in your daily life that offer a long view? It might be the top floor of a parking garage. It might be a bridge that goes over a highway or a river. It might be a specific park known for its views. Identify your personal horizon spots and visit them regularly. For one of my patients, a frontline nurse, her horizon spot was the highest point in her neighborhood. She made a ritual of parking her car there after a stressful shift and watching the sun sink behind the distant hills before heading home. She called it her emotional rinse cycle.

Mission 5: Create an Awe Inventory

The Objective: This final mission is a cognitive-behavioral tool designed to train your brain to notice and recall experiences of awe. By doing so, you are strengthening the neural pathways associated with wonder, connection, and perspective, while weakening the pathways of the overactive, self-referential Default Mode Network. You are building a personal library of antidotes to your own anxiety.

The Protocol: Your Personal Collection of Wonder

Get a Notebook: This can be part of your main Outdoor Rx journal or a separate, small notebook dedicated only to this practice.

The Prompt: At the end of each day, or once a week, take five minutes to answer this question: "What was one moment this week that made me feel small in the best possible way?"

Record the Moment: Write it down. Be specific. It doesn't have to be a grand, epic event. The power of this practice lies in learning to notice the small, everyday moments of awe that we so often miss.

Add Sensory Detail: Don't just write "I saw a sunset." Describe it. "The clouds were on fire, a deep magenta that bled into orange. It made the whole city glow for about five minutes."

Keep this List Nearby: Keep your Awe Inventory by your bed or on your desk. When feeling overwhelmed or trapped in a loop of worry, read through it. It is a powerful reminder of a larger, more beautiful reality.

Creative Examples from an Urban Awe Inventory:

- The sheer, vertical scale of a skyscraper glinting in the afternoon sun.

- The detailed, geometric perfection of a spiderweb beaded with dew on a fire escape.
- The collective, focused energy of a crowd listening to a musician in the subway.
- The surprising power of a thunderstorm seen from a high-rise window.
- The impossible number of stars that suddenly became visible during a brief city-wide power outage.

The Final Step: Make It Contagious

Awe makes us want to connect. So, the final part of this mission is to share it. Share one of your awe moments with someone else. Ask them for one of theirs. You will be amazed at the conversations this simple exchange can spark. Awe is contagious, and in spreading it, you amplify its healing power for both yourself and your community.

Nature Notes & Doctor It Up!

You now have the Sea, Sky, and Space mission parameters and guided protocols. You understand the science of why looking up and out is such a potent form of medicine for your mind, your eyes, and your nervous system. Now, as your expert coach, I want to provide you with the advanced field guide, integrating these prescriptions into the fabric of your real, often messy, modern life.

I remember standing barefoot on a massive, sun-bleached driftwood log at Refugio State Beach, a place I've visited for years near my home in Santa Barbara. The low tide revealed a wide expanse of wet, reflective sand. The sky seemed to merge seamlessly with the sea at the horizon. My mind just moments before had been a cluttered file cabinet of patient worries, farm logistics, and writing deadlines. But standing there, looking out at the sheer scale, that internal chatter unwound by itself. The sky and sea did not demand my productivity or my attention; they just offered scale, perspective, and a healthy rhythm I was missing.

This is the medicine I have prescribed more times than I can count. For the burned-out executive, the overwhelmed caregiver, the hyper-concerned parent, the anxious student, the insomniac, the prescription is often the same: "Go watch and listen to the ocean for 10 minutes." "Go find a place where you can see the sunset." "Go lie on the grass and look at the stars."

I've watched tech entrepreneurs who live their lives in hyper-vigilance finally start breathing again after 10 minutes by the Pacific Ocean. I've seen the physical difference a horizon can make in a person's posture. I see it in tourists who visit my farm in Santa Barbara, no matter where they're from, because the shift isn't subtle. It's somatic. Shoulders hunched up around the ears begin to drop. Brows furrowed in concentration begin to unfurl. This is your body responding to the powerful, non-verbal cues of vastness, safety, and scale.

Nature Note: The Magnitude of Light

Here's a reminder about the power of light: the difference between indoor and outdoor light is staggering. Recall that your typical office lighting measures about 300-500 lux. But on even the most overcast day? You're still bathing in 1000-2500 lux, so you may need to stay outside a little longer to get the benefit. A clear, sunny day delivers 10,000-25,000 lux or more.

Your brain's light sensors-those specialized cells we discussed-literally cannot distinguish between artificial twilight and complete darkness when it comes to your circadian rhythm. No wonder we feel so disconnected from natural time when we live under artificial lighting. Typical office fluorescents produce only 300-500 lux: a gap so wide that your circadian system reads the office as perpetual dusk.

Nature Note: The Overview Effect Phenomenon

Astronauts describe something called the Overview Effect. It's a cognitive shift that occurs when viewing Earth from space. They report feeling awe, a sense of unity with all life, and a dramatic reduction in personal conflicts and anxieties.

But you don't need to leave the planet to experience this. The same neurological mechanisms activate when you gaze at a vast horizon, watch clouds move across an enormous sky, or contemplate the night stars.

Your brain, confronted with true scale, automatically shifts into what researchers call broad, associative thinking. You literally see the bigger picture, not just visually, but cognitively and emotionally as well. This is why a simple sunset can solve problems that hours of rumination cannot touch.

Doctor It Up! #1: Weather as Your Mood Medicine

Start using weather as active therapy. Each type of sky offers a different neurological gift:

Stormy Skies: The dramatic contrast of dark clouds against bright breaks creates maximum visual stimulation for your awe circuits. Negative ions generated by lightning and moving water are natural mood elevators. Stand safely under cover and watch the power display. Your sympathetic nervous system gets a healthy, controlled activation. It's like a natural energy drink.

Overcast Days: That soft, diffused light is perfect for reducing visual stress and calming an overstimulated nervous system. The even illumination eliminates harsh shadows and glare, creating ideal conditions for gentle observation and reflection.

Clear Blue Infinity: This is your maximum dose of perspective medicine. The endless depth of a cloudless sky provides the strongest trigger for awe and perhaps the most effective visual reset for screen-strained eyes.

Doctor It Up! #2: The Strategic Screen Break Revolution

Repurpose your screen breaks from scrolling into doses of visual medicine. Set your phone to remind you every hour with the message "Horizon Check." When it buzzes, take 60 seconds to find the farthest point you can see through a window, from a doorway, or ideally, stepping outside. Just look.

Watercooler Fact:

Acoustic Water Bandwidth

Water sounds at **50–60 dB** create a subconscious "acoustic cocoon" that lowers heart rate and BP.

This micro-dose of distance vision is a neurological pattern interrupt. It breaks the hypnotic trance of digital tunnel vision. Subjects who use hourly horizon checks report dramatic reductions in headaches and end-of-day mental fatigue.

Doctor It Up! #3: Water Sound as Stress Medicine

Even indirect nature exposure, like water sounds, can produce restorative cognitive effects. The frequency of natural water sounds like ocean waves, babbling brooks and gentle rain falls within what acoustics researchers call the healing range of 50-15,000 Hz. These frequencies naturally slow heart rate, lower blood pressure, and shift brainwaves toward alpha and theta states associated with deep relaxation and creativity.

But here's the key: volume matters. Play water sounds at just below the level of normal conversation (about 50-60 decibels). Too loud, and it becomes stimulating rather than soothing. Too quiet, and it lacks therapeutic impact. The sweet spot creates what sound therapists call an acoustic cocoon: a gentle environment that masks jarring noises while promoting calm.

Nature Exposure vs. Blood Pressure Reduction

Research shows that regular exposure to natural enviornments can significantly reduce blood pressure levels, with benefits increasing with more time spent in nature.

The data demonstrates a clear dose-response relationship: doubling weekly nature exposure from 30 to 60 minutes increases blood pressure reduction by 40% while quadrupling exposure to 120 minutes doubles health benefit

Doctor It Up! #4: The Color Blue Prescription

Blue has measurable physiological effects. Exposure to blue environments (water, sky, blue-painted walls) can lower cortisol production, reduce heart rate, and even decrease pain perception. But reward-driven activities and artificial blue light from screens have the opposite effect, stimulating alertness and stress hormones. The difference? Natural blue light is part of a full spectrum and is reflected rather than emitted. Artificial blue light is isolated and projected directly into your retinas. To maximize your blue healing, seek natural blue environments during the day (sky, water) and reduce artificial blue light in the evening (bright screens, LED bulbs) before bed.

Blue light has nuances at night, interestingly: what you do on the screen matters as much as the glow itself. The greater danger lies in mental and cognitive arousal: sharp, bright screens and the stimulating nature of scrolling and texting emphasize the disruptive effects of blue light. But familiar, more gentle content, viewed in dim light, may even quiet rumination, even when viewed on a screen.

Doctor It Up! #5: Advanced Stargazing for Sleep

Want to supercharge your evening wind-down? Make stargazing your transition ritual between day and night.

Begin your night sky session 60-90 minutes before your target bedtime. The combination of darkness, the neck position (slightly tilted back), and the meditative quality of sky-watching creates perfect conditions for melatonin production. The gentle neck extension actually activates your parasympathetic nervous system. That's the same reason that certain yoga poses are so relaxing.

End your session by coming indoors and immediately dimming all lights. Your eyes, already adapted to darkness, will stay in night mode, preserving your body's natural preparation for sleep.

Doctor It Up! #6: Urban Sky Hunting Strategies

City dwellers aren't doomed to sky deprivation. Become a strategic urban sky hunter:

The Rooftop Revolution: Many urban apartments and office buildings have roof access. A 20-story building puts you above most light pollution and opens up dramatic sky views. Check with building management: many have policies allowing roof access during daylight hours.

Bridge Therapy: Urban bridges offer some of the best views of the sky and water in any city. Walk or drive slowly, safely. The elevation and open sightlines provide instant perspective medicine.

Reflection Doubling: Still water doubles your sky dose by creating mirror images. Urban ponds, calm sections of rivers, and even large puddles after rain can repaint a small patch of visible sky into an immersive overhead and underfoot sky experience.

The Airport Revelation: Airport observation areas and parking garages offer some of the most dramatic urban sky views available. The wide-open spaces designed for aircraft visibility create perfect horizon-watching venues.

Doctor It Up! #7: Partnering with Your Doctor: Integrating Outdoor Rx into Your Healthcare Plan

I think of Outdoor Rx as part of whole-person care, not a replacement for most medical treatment. If you speak with your doctor, ask about specifics: what do you think of 15 minutes of morning light daily? Will walking in the park after work help my blood pressure? Will two hours daily change my myopia prescription (you may know the answers, and she may not; show them the references in this book!). Ask how these practices interact with your medications and conditions. Your clinician can help tailor your medication dose and follow-up so nature and medicine work together.

Doctor It Up! #8: Tracking Your Healthspan: Advanced Metrics for Long-Term Outdoor Rx Benefits

If you like data, track trends, not single days. Wearables can show HRV and sleep stages (deep/REM) improving as your nervous system steadies. Periodic labs with your clinician (specifically Vitamin D levels, HbA1c, fasting insulin, and hs-CRP) offer another lens on inflammation, metabolism, and recovery.

Explore telomere (see Glossary) testing, epigenetic analysis to look at methylation-based organ clocks, and NAD+ levels with a specialist. VO_2 max remains the gold standard for predicting cardiorespiratory fitness and healthy years ahead, but it drops with chronic sleep loss. Even natural walking speed predicts healthspan better than most blood tests. Use metrics as feedback, not a fixation: the goal is a calmer, stronger system that holds over months and years.

Nature Note: The Seasonal Sky Prescription

Each season offers its own unique sky medicine, and your body's needs change with the light patterns:

Spring Skies: Rapid weather changes create dynamic cloud formations perfect for practicing soft fascination. Increased daylight helps reset circadian rhythms after winter.

Prescription: Cloud-watching during the dramatic weather transitions.

Summer Skies: Maximum light availability and the longest days offer peak Vitamin D synthesis and circadian anchoring. But the intensity can be overwhelming for anxious systems.

Prescription: Early morning and golden hour sky sessions, avoiding midday intensity.

Autumn Skies: The crisp air and changing atmospheric conditions create some of the year's most dramatic sunrises and sunsets. Shortening days naturally prepare your body for rest. Prescription: Sunset-watching as a daily wind-down ritual.

Winter Skies: Limited light makes every photon precious. Bare trees reveal more of the sky, while snow amplifies the available light. Prescription: Maximize all available daylight hours and embrace the dramatic contrasts of winter landscapes.

Doctor It Up! #9: The Awe Amplification Technique

To maximize the awe response from any sky experience, use this Awe Amplification protocol:

Step 1: Scale Realization. Actively contemplate the actual size of what you're observing. That cloud might be three miles tall. The moon is 240,000 miles away. Those stars are millions of times larger than Earth.

Step 2: Time Traveling. Consider the age of what you're seeing. Starlight has traveled for years, or perhaps centuries, to reach your eyes. You're literally looking backward in time.

Step 3: Connection Acknowledgment. Recognize that you are physically part of what you're observing. The calcium in your bones was forged in the heart of an ancient star. You are the universe becoming aware of itself.

This technique changes casual observation into a deep experience, maximizing the Default Mode Network reset we discussed in the science section.

Doctor It Up! #10: Emergency Awe Protocol

For acute anxiety or overwhelm, this rapid-response technique can interrupt panic cycles:

The 5-4-3-2-1 Sky Reset:

- 5 things you can see in the sky (clouds, birds, contrails, etc.)
- 4 qualities of light you notice (brightness, color, direction, shadows)
- 3 sounds from the environment around you
- 2 physical sensations (air temperature, wind, sun warmth)
- 1 slow, deep breath while maintaining sky contact

This grounds you in your senses while providing the perspective medicine of looking up and out. It can stop a panic attack in its tracks by engaging your observational mind and breaking the internal spiral.

A Final Diagnostic Tool

As a physician, I have learned that sometimes the most powerful questions are the simplest. If you want to understand the state of someone's connection to the natural world, or your own, try asking this:

"When was the last time you watched the sky do something?"

The answer is often more revealing than a full medical history. It is both a diagnostic tool and a suggested prescription. People who regularly watch sunrises, cloud movements, star patterns, and weather changes have measurably lower stress levels, better sleep quality, and enhanced cognitive flexibility. They literally maintain a broader perspective on life's challenges.

The sky is always doing something. The question is: are you paying attention?

Your Outdoor Rx Action Space: The Horizon Log & Awe Inventory

These prompts are designed to help you actively practice the art of looking up and out. This is your dedicated space to train your perception, document your discoveries, and build a personal library of awe and perspective.

Try setting aside one analog afternoon each week with no texts, no scrolling and just face-to-face time in the real world. That could mean a stroll through a local market, a picnic at the lake, writing a letter by hand, or even a no-tech board game night. These moments may seem small, but they compound into deeper trust, sharper presence, and more grounded connection.

In a culture that prizes speed and spectacle, this is how you begin to reclaim real human closeness, one unplugged hour at a time. Use an Outdoor Rx notebook to create your Horizon Log. This is not a chore; it is an act of reclaiming your attention and your sense of place in the universe.

Your Mission Prompts

Become a Horizon Hunter: Your first task is to identify your personal horizon spots. Name at least three places in or near your neighborhood where you can see a wide, expansive view. This could be a park hill, a rooftop you have access to, a beach, a bridge over a highway, or the top floor of a public parking garage. List them here.

___

Schedule a Sky Break: Look at your calendar for the coming week right now. Find one 15-minute slot and schedule a firmly set appointment with yourself labeled Sky Break. When the time comes, go to one of your horizon spots and simply watch the sky or the water.

Curate Your Auditory Sanctuary: Download a nature sound app (like Calm or myNoise) or find a high-quality, long-form recording of a natural soundscape on YouTube. Choose one sound like ocean waves, gentle rain, or wind in the pines and commit to playing it as a daily transition ritual (e.g., for the first five minutes of your lunch break, or while you brush your teeth before bed).

The Sky, Twice a Day: Once this week, take a photograph of the same patch of sky from the same spot in the morning and again in the evening. Put the two photos side-by-side. Notice the significant shifts in color, light, and mood. Share the two photos with a friend and ask which one they are drawn to more.

Journal Your Experience: After your first Sky Break, spend five minutes writing in your journal in response to this simple prompt: "How does looking at the vastness of the sky make me feel in my body?"

Spread the Awe: Ask someone you love this question: What's your favorite memory involving water? Listen to their story. Sharing these experiences is a powerful form of connection.

Create a Micro-Cue: Take a small sticky note and write three words on it: LOOK UP TODAY. Tape it to the corner of your bathroom mirror or your computer monitor. Let it be your gentle, daily reminder to break the downward gaze and connect with the scale of the world above and beyond you.

Chapter 3: Forest-Bathing Rx: Inhale Immunity, Reset Your Nervous System

Introduction: Enter the Forest, Heal from the Inside Out

Is your mind a runaway train? A clattering whirlwind of to-do lists, anxious what-ifs, and the endless ping of digital alerts? Do you feel a weariness deep in your bones that sleep can't touch? If that sounds familiar, you are not alone.

You're battling the Indoor Epidemic head-on, and frankly, you're exhausted. Your nervous system is on high alert, marinating in a low-grade bath of stress hormones. If you are crying out for a genuine reset a way to unwind the tightly coiled tension in your soul-then it's time to engage with what this chapter offers.

You're about to unleash nature's secret weapon for cellular defense and mental clarity! When you breathe in the forest, you're literally inhaling phytoncides, which are aromatic compounds trees release that supercharge your immune system by dramatically boosting your Natural Killer (NK) cells (see Glossary).

> **Watercooler Fact:**
>
> Forest Pharmacy: A single two-hour forest bath increases your cancer-fighting NK cells by 56% and the effect lasts 30 days.

These NK cells are like the Navy SEALs of your immune system: an important type of white blood cell that serves as your body's elite special forces, tasked with seeking and destroying virally infected cells and, importantly, the early surveillance and elimination of nascent tumor cells before they can become full-blown cancer.

Think about this: just one forest session can give you a month of enhanced immune protection, a direct upgrade to your healthspan.

Beyond that, nature's soft fascination is like plugging your brain in, allowing your overtaxed attention to rest and recover for measurable cognitive gains. Here's a mind-blower: a 90-minute walk in nature slashes rumination by calming the subgenual prefrontal cortex (the brain area tied to anxiety and depression) giving you a direct cognitive upgrade.

And get this: you don't even have to love the walk to get these brain and attention benefits. Studies show it works just as well in freezing weather as on a perfect day, proving it's a deep physiological effect, not just a mood boost. These good feelings counter negative emotions that hasten decline and deliver small but powerful boosts to your overall well-being and health, and longevity.

This is your prescription for Forest-Bathing Rx. This is how you turn your 7% into a dose of nature-based medicine.

The Japanese call it Shinrin-Yoku, translated as forest bathing. But this isn't about getting wet. It's about what happens when you stop moving like you're late for everything and start moving like the trees are trying to tell you something.

Which they are, both through the tree aromas and fractal patterns that make your overstimulated brain exhale in relief. Trees have a sensory intelligence that puts your smartphone to shame: not because the device can't connect you, but because it doesn't know how to feel. The art of being fully present and receptive is practiced in forest bathing, and it too is an antidote to the list-filled pace that defines and depletes modern life.

This practice emerged from Japan in the 1980s as their own SOS response to the Indoor Epidemic. Japanese researchers were watching their people literally work themselves to death. They even coined a term for it: karoshi, meaning death from overwork. The government stepped in and commissioned studies to understand how contact with nature could serve as preventive medicine. What they discovered was nothing short of revolutionary, changing everything we know about the therapeutic power of the natural world.

The Japanese approach to Shinrin-Yoku is brilliantly anti-achievement. There are no fitness goals, no summit to conquer, no calories to burn. Instead, the entire focus is on what they call taking in the forest atmosphere, a specific shift in pace and intention that distinguishes it from traditional exercise. In Japan, forest bathing is now prescribed by doctors and covered by health insurance. Forests are designated as forest therapy bases with trained guides and specific protocols for different health conditions.

The research is so compelling that countries around the world are scrambling to create their own forest-therapy programs. Measurable changes in stress hormones, immune function, brain activity, and cardiovascular health are just the beginning. Forest bathing doesn't just help you feel better; it actually makes your body better and begins to heal it at a cellular level.

The Why: Your Science Snapshot

The Crucial Distinction: Why This Isn t Exercise

Let me be clear: Forest bathing is NOT just a walk in the woods. It's not about step counts or conquering peaks. It's a deliberate slowing down and a direct defiance of our always-on culture and it's where real healing happens. A hike often has a goal, such as the summit, a waterfall, or a step count. Your mind is laser-focused on navigation and achievement. Your heart rate is pumping, your breathing is labored, and your attention is split between the physical challenge and the destination ahead.

Watercooler Fact:

Forest Parasympathetic Switch
Forest bathing activates deep parasympathetic recovery through sensory slowing not exertion.

Forest bathing throws all that out the window. It has no destination. The entire point is the journey or, more accurately, abandoning the journey for pure presence. It's an absurdly slow, meandering pace with frequent, intentional pauses. You aren't stopping because you're tired; you're stopping to absorb the world. Your heart rate should decrease, not increase. Your breathing should deepen and slow. Your attention should become completely absorbed in the immediate sensory experience of where you are right now.

Think of it this way: you can chug a glass of wine to quench thirst, or you can sip it slowly, noticing its color, aroma, and complex flavors. Both meet the goal of consuming wine, but only one provides a rich, multi-sensory experience that engages your entire nervous system. Forest bathing is the sensory sipping of the natural world.

This distinction matters because your nervous system responds completely differently to these two approaches. Goal-oriented outdoor activity, while beneficial, keeps your sympathetic nervous system engaged. You're still in doing mode, still achieving, still pushing toward an outcome. Forest bathing specifically targets the parasympathetic nervous system, your body's rest and digest mode. It's the perfect antidote to our achievement-obsessed culture, not another item to add to your performance checklist.

The Japanese research is crystal clear about this. Participants who forest bathed showed dramatic decreases in stress hormones and increases in relaxation markers. Participants who hiked the same trails at a normal pace showed minimal changes or even increases in stress markers despite the physical exercise benefits. The pace and intention completely flip the physiological script.

> **Watercooler Fact:**
> Rumination Reduction: A 90-minute nature walk significantly reduces activity in the brain region linked to depression and anxiety.

You must slow down to receive the medicine. This is perhaps the most challenging part for people accustomed to squeezing productivity out of every moment. Every instinct will scream at you to walk faster, cover more ground, and make the most of your outdoor time. These instincts are precisely what you're healing from. The slowing down *is* the medicine.

The Stress-Busting Cascade: Taming Your Runaway Nervous System

One of forest bathing's most powerful effects is on your stress response. When you dedicate some of your 7% to forest bathing, you're hitting the reset button on your stress response. For a nervous system stuck in fight-or-flight mode, this is your frontline therapy.

Let me tell you about David, a dedicated high school history teacher who came to my clinic with chronic tension headaches that were ruling his life. They would start at the base of his skull and wrap around his head like a medieval torture device, getting progressively worse throughout the school day. He was also irritable, had trouble sleeping, and felt constant tension in his shoulders and jaw.

David was a textbook case of a nervous system stuck in sympathetic overdrive. The constant demands of managing a classroom full of teenagers had his body in a perpetual state of low-grade fight or flight. His nervous system was treating every school day like a war zone, flooding his system with stress hormones from the moment his alarm went off until well into the evening.

During our initial consultation, David described feeling tired but wired-exhausted but unable to truly relax. This state was a direct result of chronic stress.

His body was running on empty and his cortisol was still high in the evening, blocking melatonin--the hormone that should have been preparing him for sleep. He'd come home from school physically drained but mentally agitated, unable to shift gears from teacher mode to human mode. His wife had commented that he seemed always braced for the next crisis, even during peaceful moments at home. This is textbook chronic stress syndrome, a nervous system that has forgotten how to downshift.

The Hormonal Cascade of Chronic Stress

Let's talk cortisol, the primary activity hormone that's probably coursing through your veins right now. In healthy patterns, cortisol follows a natural rhythm: high in the morning to help you wake up and face the day, then gradually declining throughout the day to prepare your body for restorative sleep. A morning pulse is healthy and necessary. However, chronically elevated cortisol, the kind that results from unremitting stress like David's, is like having acid rain inside your body.

Chronically elevated cortisol is a destroyer. It disrupts sleep by interfering with melatonin production. It impairs cognitive function by attacking the hippocampus, the brain region crucial for memory formation. It promotes weight gain, particularly dangerous visceral fat around the midsection, by triggering cravings for high-calorie foods and slowing metabolism. It suppresses immune function by reducing the production and effectiveness of infection-fighting white blood cells. It contributes to insulin resistance, setting the stage for diabetes. It promotes inflammation (see Glossary) throughout the body, accelerating aging and increasing cardiovascular risk. Chronic cortisol elevation is literally aging you from the inside out, and it's happening right now.

Here's where forest bathing becomes your secret weapon: it tames runaway cortisol with remarkable effectiveness. Multiple studies have consistently shown that sensory immersion in a forest environment leads to significant decreases in salivary and urinary cortisol levels. We're talking about lowering cortisol levels by as much as 21% beyond the normal daily variation.

Stop and think about that for a moment. This isn't just a subjective feeling of relaxation; it's a measurable, physiological shift in your stress hormone profile. You are literally washing stress from your system. The practice also reduces levels of adrenaline and noradrenaline, the other key fight-or-flight hormones that keep your system revved like a race car engine.

How Nature Signals Safety

The mechanism behind this cortisol reduction is fascinating and reveals why artificial stress-reduction techniques often fall flat. A safe natural environment usually offers complex, non-threatening and multi-sensory inputs. Some of these are the gentle, non-rhythmic sounds of birdsong and wind, earthy smells and soft, filtered light. They all send a powerful, coherent safety signal to the most ancient parts of your brain.

Your amygdala, the brain's alarm system, constantly scans your environment for threats, much like a hypervigilant security guard. In modern life, it's overwhelmed by signals that trigger low-level alarm: the harsh angles of buildings, the constant noise of traffic, the blue light of screens, and the chemical smells of urban environments. These signals keep your nervous system in a state of subtle but persistent arousal, like being stuck in a perpetual state of stage fright.

Natural environments provide the opposite input. The organic curves and patterns found in nature are inherently soothing to our visual processing systems. The complex but harmonious soundscapes of forests provide pink noise, described previously as a frequency distribution that promotes relaxation and mental clarity. The scents of plants and earth trigger positive associations stored deep in our evolutionary memory. These inputs combine to tell your nervous system that there is no immediate threat, that it is safe to stand down from high alert.

David's Transformation

I prescribed David a specific protocol: a slow, 45-minute walk in a local wooded park three times a week after school. The timing was important and right after his most stressful part of the day, when his cortisol levels were highest. I gave him specific instructions to leave his phone in the car, to walk at what would feel like an almost absurdly slow pace, and to focus on the sensory practices you'll learn in the How-To section.

The park David chose wasn't some majestic wilderness: just a five-acre wooded area with paved paths, maintained by the city parks department. But it had mature oak and maple trees, a small creek, and enough distance from the road that traffic noise faded into the background. Most importantly, it was a 14-minute drive from his school, making it accessible even on his most chaotic days.

The first week was rough. David reported feeling antsy and kept catching himself walking too fast, mentally planning lessons, or worrying about the next day's classes. This is normal. An overstimulated nervous system doesn't immediately know how to relax. It's like a car engine that's been revving at high RPMs for hours. It takes time to drop down to idle, and the engine's timing probably needs to be recalibrated.

But by week two, something shifted. David began to notice that his drive home from the park felt different. The usual mental chatter about school problems was quieter. He arrived home, actually present for dinner conversations with his wife, rather than physically there but mentally still in his classroom.

By the six-week mark, David's life changes were clear to everyone around him. His wife commented that he seemed like himself again. His students noticed that Mr. Peterson was more patient and had a sense of humor that had been missing. David, himself reported that he was sleeping better than he had in years and felt a sense of resilience he'd forgotten was possible.

> **Watercooler Fact:**
>
> 5-Minute Green Lift: Spending as little as five minutes in green space measurably boosts mood and self-esteem, with the biggest effects occurring the fastest.

The Nervous System Rebalance: Understanding HRV

This rebalance is measured objectively by Heart Rate Variability (HRV) (see Glossary), which serves as a report card for your nervous system and a proxy for your stress level. HRV measures the subtle variations in the time intervals between your heartbeats. Contrary to what you might expect, a healthy heart doesn't beat like a metronome with perfectly regular intervals. Instead, it constantly makes tiny changes in response to your breathing, thoughts, emotions, and environment.

A high HRV indicates a nervous system that's flexible, resilient, and able to adapt quickly to changing demands. HRV reflects your autonomic nervous system, which has a sympathetic (aka fight-or-flight) branch and a parasympathetic (aka rest-and-digest) branch. A low HRV suggests a system that's stuck, inflexible, and struggling to adapt and recover from modern demands.

Forest bathing consistently boosts HRV, strengthening the parasympathetic brake that allows your body to heal and recover. The range of everyday HRVs can be wide and vary significantly from one person to another. Personal tracking is valuable for understanding your own patterns over time. Studies using HRV monitors have shown that just 15 minutes of mindful time in nature can significantly and helpfully increase HRV, with effects lasting for hours after the experience ends.

The vagus nerve makes forest bathing physiologic. Nature's steady safety signals (sound, light, scent, touch, trusted company) strengthen your stress thermostat and reset the system that governs stress, mood, immunity, and digestion. The Outdoor Rx sequences ahead are built to tune that pathway, simply and repeatedly.

When David practiced his slow, mindful walks, he was retraining his nervous system. He was teaching it, through embodied experience, how to access a state of calm. His reduced headaches resulted directly from his neck and shoulder muscles finally receiving the signal to release their chronic tension.

Nature's Pharmacy: The Hidden Chemical Communication

But here's where the science goes from impressive to mind-blowing. This is where forest bathing transcends simple relaxation. Trees and plants, to protect themselves from being eaten by insects or infected by bacteria and fungi, produce and release phytoncides (see Glossary), which you now know are a complex array of airborne aromatic compounds, and literally mean plant-derived exterminators.

These compounds are fundamentally the plant's own sophisticated, natural immune system. They include familiar wood essential oils such as alpha-pinene (which gives pine trees their characteristic scent), d-limonene (found in citrus), beta-pinene, camphene, and many others. Each tree species produces its own unique cocktail of these protective compounds, creating what some researchers call the chemical fingerprint of different forests.

When you breathe in forest air, you're not just catching the scent of pine. You're inhaling a living pharmacy.

Phytoncides like alpha pinene and limonene move through your nose and lungs and begin changing activity inside your cells. They boost your calming GABA circuits. They quiet NF kappa B, the pathway that drives inflammation. They protect neurons from oxidative stress and even act as direct antioxidants.

These compounds reach the brain's immune sentries, the microglia, and help settle them down. That shift reduces the background noise of inflammation and allows your nervous system to step out of fight or flight. The result is a clear signal for repair. Your body and mind finally get the chance to recover.

At the same time, your immune special forces (NK cells, as described previously) take off and sweep for viruses and rogue cancer cells. The result: lower cortisol levels, a steadier mood, sharper focus, and less of the slow burn of chronic inflammation that accelerates aging. This is cellular reprogramming. Every deep breath among trees is a reminder that longevity doesn't begin with another pill. It begins with air charged by living forests.

The Groundbreaking Research of Dr. Qing Li

When we walk through a forest and breathe in the air, we inhale these phytoncides. Groundbreaking research by Dr. Qing Li, an immunologist at the Nippon Medical School in Tokyo, has shown that inhaling these natural compounds triggers a significant and lasting boost in our own immune function.

Dr. Li's research began with a simple but intriguing observation: people living in areas with more forest coverage had lower rates of cancer. This led him to investigate whether there might be a direct connection between forest exposure and immune function. What he discovered was extraordinary and completely changed our understanding of the relationship between nature and human health.

Specifically, Dr. Li's studies have shown that forest bathing leads to a dramatic increase in both the number and, crucially, the functional activity of our robust and active NK cell population, which is absolutely crucial for a healthy immune system. When NK cells are functioning optimally, they provide constant surveillance against viral infections, help prevent autoimmune disorders, and serve as your first line of defense against cancer development.

The Remarkable Study Results

In one of his most cited studies, Dr. Li took a group of office workers, people with lifestyle profiles much like ours, on a three-day, two-night forest-bathing trip. These weren't athletes or health enthusiasts; they were regular people dealing with regular urban stresses and probably spending way too much time staring at screens. He measured their NK cell activity before the trip, right after, and then again seven days and 30 days later.

The results were astounding. After the forest trip, the participants' NK cell activity increased by over 50%. This wasn't just a temporary boost like you might get from a cup of green tea. The immune enhancement was sustained and powerful. Even more, this powerful immune-boosting effect remained significantly elevated a full 30 days after they had returned to the city. A single forest-bathing experience provided enhanced immune protection for a month. Let me repeat that: one weekend in the forest gave them 30 days of boosted immunity.

Dr. Li then conducted controlled experiments to isolate the mechanism. He exposed people to phytoncides in laboratory settings, with no other forest elements present, and found that the phytoncides alone were sufficient to boost NK cell activity. He identified the most effective compounds and measured optimal concentrations for immune enhancement.

This research has been replicated in multiple countries with consistent results. Studies in South Korea, Finland, and Germany have all confirmed that forest bathing leads to measurable improvements in immune function. This isn't about feeling good; it's about tangibly enhancing your body's ability to defend itself at a cellular level.

Your Personal Immune-Boosting Session

When you practice forest bathing, you are not just taking in fresh oxygen; you are literally inhaling nature's own complex, immune-support pharmacy that has been refined over millions of years of evolution. Every breath in a forest delivers thousands of these protective compounds directly to your lungs, where they enter your bloodstream and begin their immune-enhancing work.

Certain trees are potent sources of immune-boosting phytoncides. Coniferous trees, such as pine, fir, cedar, cypress, and spruce, are absolute phytoncide powerhouses. The Japanese Hinoki cypress, used in traditional Japanese architecture specifically for its antimicrobial properties, releases some of the most potent immune-enhancing compounds, especially Hinokitiol. Citrus and juniper trees are rich in limonene, which is known for its antidepressant effects. Clove and hemp emit beta-caryophyllene, which acts through the endocannabinoid pathway.

Phytoncides are fundamentally forest aromatherapy but stronger, because they evolved with us. The concentration of these tree aromas varies with weather conditions, so you can actually optimize your exposure. Humid days, especially after rain, tend to have higher concentrations of these compounds. Early morning and evening usually have the highest concentrations of phytoncides. This is why many forest-bathing practitioners report that misty, slightly damp conditions often provide the deepest experiences.

The Cognitive Upgrade: Restoring Your Mental Firepower

In our age of fractured attention and digital overwhelm, forest bathing offers a direct cognitive upgrade and a system restore for your brain. The attention-restoration benefits are primarily explained by Attention Restoration Theory, developed by environmental psychologists Rachel and Stephen Kaplan after decades of research on how different environments affect cognitive function.

Understanding Your Two Types of Attention

We have two main types of attention, and understanding this distinction is important to grasping why forest bathing is so cognitively restorative and why you feel so mentally fried at the end of most days:

Directed Attention: This is the focused, effortful attention we use for work, studying, driving in heavy traffic, reading dense material, and navigating our digital devices. It's voluntary, requires serious mental effort, and can be fatigued with overuse, like any muscle that's worked too hard. Think of it as your brain's high-beam headlights, powerful and focused, but with limited battery life.

When directed attention becomes fatigued, you experience what researchers call mental fatigue or cognitive overload. You might notice difficulty concentrating, increased irritability, impaired decision-making, and a general feeling of mental fog. You've literally exhausted your brain's ability to maintain focused attention, and as you're reading this, there's a good chance you're there right now.

Involuntary Attention (or Soft Fascination): This is an effortless, bottom-up form of attention captured by inherently interesting stimuli in our environment. It doesn't require conscious effort and actually helps restore your capacity for directed attention, like letting your overworked muscles rest while still staying active.

The key insight is that natural environments are filled with stimuli that evoke soft fascination. Think of the gentle rustling of leaves, the dance of light and shadow on the forest floor, the meandering flight of a butterfly, the complex, ever-changing patterns of clouds moving across the sky, or the rhythmic sound of waves or flowing water.

These natural phenomena are interesting enough to hold our attention gently, but they don't demand our full cognitive effort. Unlike hard fascination (like watching an action movie or playing a video game), which can be mentally exhausting despite being engaging, soft fascination is inherently restorative, like a mental massage.

The Science of Mental Restoration

This state of soft fascination allows your depleted directed-attention muscles to rest and recover. It's like putting your brain on a charger while keeping it engaged. Multiple studies have shown this restoration effect with measurable cognitive improvements that would make any nootropic supplement envious.

A landmark study by Berman and his colleagues showed that a 50-minute walk in a park improved performance on a demanding attention task by 20% compared to a walk of the same duration on a busy city street. The urban walk showed no cognitive improvement and sometimes even slight decreases in performance due to the mental effort required to navigate traffic, noise, and urban stimuli.

Breaking the Rumination Cycle

Forest bathing also directly tackles one of the most cognitively destructive habits of modern life: rumination. Rumination is that toxic mental pattern of getting stuck in repetitive, negative thought loops about ourselves, our problems, our past mistakes, or our future worries. It's the mental equivalent of a car stuck in a ditch, spinning its wheels deeper and deeper into the same rut, and it's absolutely exhausting.

Using fMRI, researchers at Stanford University found that a 90-minute walk in a natural setting significantly reduced activity in the subgenual prefrontal cortex. This brain region is highly active during rumination and is strongly linked to the risk for depression and anxiety disorders.

Participants who walked for the same duration in an urban environment showed no reduction in this brain activity. Some showed slight increases, suggesting that urban environments might actually promote rumination rather than reduce it, adding insult to injury.

The mechanism seems to be that the rich, multi-sensory details of the natural world naturally draw our attention outward, away from our internal mental chatter. When you're genuinely absorbed in watching the way light filters through leaves or listening to the layered complexity of forest sounds, your brain literally doesn't have the resources to run anxious thought loops.

Sarah's Cognitive Transformation

Let me tell you about Sarah, a caregiver drowning in her city apartment while caring for her elderly mother with dementia. When Sarah first came to see me for high blood pressure, she described feeling like her brain was constantly buzzing with worry and exhaustion. She felt like a swarm of bees was living in her head. She was responsible for her mother's medications, doctor appointments, safety, and daily care while also trying to manage her own life and part-time work.

Sarah's blood pressure was high (145/95) so we treated it. But her blood pressure was not high enough to cause what she was feeling. Her buzzing was a classic sign of attention fatigue: difficulty concentrating on simple tasks, forgetting where she put things, feeling overwhelmed by basic decisions like what to make for dinner, and an inability to read or focus on anything for more than a few minutes. She described her mind as feeling scattered and said she often felt like she was "thinking through mud."

The caregiving stress had created a perfect storm for rumination. Sarah lay awake at night, cycling through worries about her mother's declining health, guilt about not being a good enough caregiver, fear about the future, and resentment about the loss of her own life.

Sarah's initial response to my suggestion of forest bathing was skeptical. "I can barely leave my mother alone for 30 minutes," she said. "How am I supposed to go to a forest?" This is when we discovered the life-changing yet accessible power of urban forest bathing.

Sarah's sanctuary became the small courtyard of her apartment complex. It had one large oak tree, a few bushes, and a patch of grass. Not exactly a forest, but it was alive and growing. The positive changes for her began with just 15 minutes in this tiny green space each morning before her mother woke up.

At first, Sarah reported that her mind was too agitated to really focus on the sensory experiences. She would sit under the oak tree and immediately plan her mother's day, worrying about upcoming doctor appointments or replaying conversations with her mother's physician. This is completely normal for someone whose nervous system has been running on high alert for months.

But I encouraged Sarah to notice when her mind wandered and gently return her attention to something in her immediate environment: the texture of the tree bark, the sound of birds, the feeling of air on her skin. Each time she noticed her mind had wandered and brought it back, she was strengthening her ability to interrupt rumination patterns. In a way, she was training her attention muscles.

Within three weeks of daily 15-minute courtyard sessions, Sarah began noticing changes that amazed her. She reported that her mind felt clearer, and that she was less likely to lose her train of thought mid-sentence. Simple tasks like organizing medications or preparing meals felt less overwhelming. Most remarkably, she slept better because the nightly worry cycles were less intense and easier to interrupt.

For Sarah, her urban courtyard became a revelation. At first, all she could hear was city noise, like traffic, sirens, neighbors. But by consciously listening to the urban sounds, she began to notice the sparrows' song in the oak trees, the wind blowing through their leaves, and the scuttling of a squirrel. She was now training her brain to find the natural signal, even above the din of the artificial noise of the city. She was trying to tune into a radio station through the static, and she started to succeed.

The cognitive benefits became apparent in her daily caregiving. Sarah found she could more easily remember her mother's care instructions, felt less scattered when managing multiple tasks, and, most important, stayed present with her mother rather than being constantly distracted by worried thoughts about the future. The 15 minutes of morning forest bathing were giving her the cognitive resources she needed to handle the demands of the rest of her day.

Within six weeks, Sarah had expanded her practice to include afternoon window forest-bathing sessions, where she would sit by her mother's bedroom window (which overlooked a small neighborhood park) and practice the same sensory awareness techniques while her mother napped. Sarah's chronic anxiety had significantly decreased, and she felt more equipped to handle the emotional demands of caregiving. The quality of her attention had improved so much that she returned to reading, something she hadn't enjoyed for months.

The Cardiovascular and Mood Revolution

> **Watercooler Fact:**
>
> **Forest Bathing Lowers BP Like a Drug**
> A single **2-hour** forest-bathing session drops SBP by **7 mmHg** and DBP by **4 mmHg**, a measurable cardiovascular dose.

The cardiovascular benefits of forest bathing are immediate and measurable. Studies consistently show that forest immersion leads to measurable reductions in both blood pressure and heart rate within just 15-20 minutes of beginning the practice. Forest bathing involves very gentle movement at a leisurely pace. The cardiovascular changes are primarily driven by nervous system shifts and the stress-hormone reductions we discussed earlier.

> **Watercooler Fact:**
>
> **The Green Blood Pressure Pill**
> Outdoor movement lowers SBP by **five mmHg**, equivalent to starting a first-line antihypertensive.

A study of middle-aged men with hypertension found that a single two-hour forest-bathing session reduced systolic blood pressure by an average of seven mmHg and diastolic pressure by four mmHg.

> **Watercooler Fact**
>
> **Nature's Stroke Shield**
> A five **mmHg** SBP drop = **14% lower stroke risk** and **9% lower heart-attack risk:** nature delivering pharmaceutical-level impact.

These reductions continued for days after the forest exposure ended. For context, a 5 mmHg reduction in systolic blood pressure is associated with a 14% reduction in stroke risk and a 9% reduction in heart attack risk. That's pharmaceutical-level effectiveness from walking slowly in the woods.

The Biochemistry of Nature-Induced Happiness

> **Watercooler Fact:**
>
> **Nature + People = Stress Melter**
> Time outside with someone raises **oxytocin**, directly countering cortisol's stress chemistry.

The mood-boosting effects of forest bathing are equally impressive. They operate through multiple biochemical pathways in the brain and the gut, resulting in both immediate and lasting improvements in emotional well-being.

Studies consistently show that forest bathing significantly reduces negative mood states such as tension, anxiety, anger, fatigue, and confusion, while simultaneously increasing positive feelings such as vigor, happiness, and awe. However, the research goes beyond subjective mood reports to measure actual changes in brain chemistry.

A study on middle-aged men in Japan found that a forest-bathing program not only increased their feelings of vigor and reduced fatigue but also led to a measurable increase in their serum serotonin levels. Serotonin is often called the "happiness neurotransmitter" because of its important role in mood regulation, sleep quality, appetite control, and overall well-being.

The serotonin boost from forest bathing seems to work through several mechanisms. Exposure to natural light, especially in the morning, helps regulate circadian rhythms and supports healthy serotonin production. The stress reduction from cortisol lowering removes an important inhibitor of serotonin synthesis. The physical act of gentle movement in nature promotes the production of brain-derived neurotrophic factor, which supports the growth and maintenance of serotonin-producing neurons.

Forest environments also promote the production of endorphins, your body's natural feel-good chemicals. These are the same compounds released during exercise, laughter, and other pleasurable activities. The difference is that forest bathing promotes endorphin release through relaxation and sensory pleasure rather than physical exertion. In a sense, you're getting a runner's high without running.

The Awe Factor

> **Watercooler Fact:**
>
> **Awe as Anti-Inflammatory Medicine**
> Looking at the horizon or sky strengthens **vagal tone** and dampens inflammation.

Awe, discussed in Chapter 2, is again that sense of wonder and connection you feel when confronted with something beautiful, vast, or intense. Forest environments are powerful generators of awe because they reveal the complexity and beauty of natural systems. Even a simple forest has millions of individual organisms working together in complex patterns that have evolved over millions of years. When we slow down enough to really perceive this complexity, it naturally evokes awe and wonder.

Forest-bathing mechanisms work together. The drop in cortisol lowers blood pressure and heart rate, and an improved mood reduces inflammation. These changes enhance recovery from stress and create a positive feedback loop that strengthens both resilience and cardiovascular function. At the same time, phytoncides boost immunity and calm the nervous system. They lower inflammatory cytokines, which are molecules such as interleukin-6 and TNF-alpha: two molecules the body makes that have been linked to worsened stress and depression.

This is why forest bathing so often feels other-worldly rather than simply relaxing: you're simultaneously activating multiple internal healing processes. The result internally is additive and synergistic.

Watercooler Fact

PTSD Forest Dose
A single **2-hour** guided forest session reduces PTSD symptoms by **18%**.

The How-To: Your Sensory Immersion Journey

Your task is to begin this fundamental, evidence-based practice for at least 30 minutes, once. For a truly deep, restorative, and potentially transformative dive, I encourage you to allow for a generous and unhurried one to two hours, or even longer if your schedule permits.

The main goal is to let go of any preconceived expectations, agendas, or specific goals you might normally bring to an outdoor excursion. Instead, your entire focus will be on the art of being fully present and gently receiving the myriad sensory experiences offered by the surrounding environment.

Phase 1: Preparation --Choosing Your Sanctuary with Care

The first step in any successful mission is reconnaissance and preparation. Choose a location that feels both safe and conducive to the practice. This is about finding your personal place of peace and sensory richness-your own little slice of healing heaven.

What to Look For: Select a safe, accessible, and appealing natural place that truly allows for quiet contemplation, slow, unhurried movement, and relatively undisturbed sensory engagement. This does not have to be some remote, old-growth forest that requires a three-day expedition to reach. A cherished local park that boasts mature trees and quiet, secluded corners can be perfect. A public botanical garden, with its diverse plantings and often peaceful pathways, can be a wonderful choice. A well-maintained forest trail, a tranquil path that meanders alongside a gently flowing river, a serene lake, or a peaceful beach can all serve as ideal sanctuaries. Even a thriving community garden, if it welcomes respectful visitors during its open hours, can offer a surprising wealth of sensory experiences.

Consider my patient Sarah, the caregiver who felt trapped in her city apartment caring for her elderly mother. Finding sanctuary first felt impossible to her. Her victory was in redefining the term. Her sanctuary became the small, often-overlooked courtyard of her apartment complex. It had one large oak tree, a few bushes, and a patch of grass. It wasn't a forest, but it was alive and breathing. She learned that the quality of your attention is infinitely more important than the grandeur of the location. Look for the pockets of nature available to you: a tree-lined street, a small pocket park, or even a single, resilient tree growing through the sidewalk. These can be potent places for this practice.

Mission Logistics: Before you head out, take a moment to plan like the strategic health warrior you are. If you're going alone, especially to a more remote or unfamiliar area, always tell someone reliable of your specific plans, including your location and expected return time. Consider bringing a bottle of water and maybe a small, lightweight mat, blanket, or cushion if you anticipate wanting to sit comfortably on the ground for extended periods. I highly encourage this in this deeply receptive practice.

Urban Forest Bathing: Your City Sanctuary

Urban forest bathing is a legitimate and powerful practice that can be extraordinarily effective precisely because you're creating an oasis of calm within the chaos. The contrast itself becomes therapeutic magic. Your nervous system experiences an even more dramatic shift when you find deep peace amid urban intensity.

The Single Tree Sanctuary: Find a tree, even a solitary specimen growing through a sidewalk crack, like nature's middle finger to concrete and make it your practice partner. Place your palm against its bark and notice the texture variations, temperature differences, and subtle vibrations you can feel. Look up into its canopy and practice tree gazing: soften your focus and watch how light moves through the leaves like a natural light show. Even street trees filter thousands of gallons of air daily and release oxygen and phytoncides. That sidewalk oak is working as hard as any forest giant.

The Pocket Park Protocol: Repurpose any small green space into a complete forest-bathing environment. A 20x20-foot patch of grass with a few shrubs contains an entire ecosystem that can be discovered if you know how to look. There's a whole universe in your backyard. Get down on hands and knees and explore the micro-landscape. Notice how many shades of green exist in just one square foot. Listen for the tiny sounds: insects moving, grass blades rustling. Pocket parks often host surprising wildlife; urban sparrows, squirrels, and even hawks frequent these spaces.

Window Forest Bathing: If outdoor access is truly limited, practice threshold forest bathing from a window. Open it and practice the listening meditation, tuning into whatever natural sounds penetrate the urban noise. Watch cloud movements with the same attention you'd give to a forest canopy if you were outside. If you can see any trees, even distant ones, practice the soft-gaze technique.

Place a small potted plant on your windowsill and tend to it as part of your practice. The act of nurturing indoor plant life provides many of the same nervous system benefits as being in larger natural spaces. This is how analog wellness begins: not with a hack, but with a small, quiet choice to protect your nervous system.

Phase 2: The Beginning --Marking the Threshold and Slowing Down Intentionally

This phase is about creating a clear and conscious transition from your ordinary state of mind to the receptive state required for forest bathing: pretend you're switching from AM radio to high-definition surround sound.

Marking the Threshold: A Conscious and Intentional Start

As you arrive at the entrance of your chosen space, pause. Do not rush in like you're late for a meeting. Stand at the edge of the trailhead, the park gate, the entrance to the garden and take a moment to mark this transition consciously. This ritual signals to your mind and body that you are shifting from your everyday routine, with its mental preoccupations and jarring demands, into a dedicated time for healing and connection.

Take three deep, slow, centering breaths that actually mean something. Let your exhale last a beat longer than your inhale. This simple pattern directly engages the vagus, lowers sympathetic drive, and improves gas exchange.

You naturally take shallow breaths when you're anxious or hunched over a screen. That activates your body's stress response, raises your blood pressure, and limits oxygen exchange. But when you take deeper breaths, starting from your diaphragm and fully expanding your lungs, you improve your posture and let more carbon dioxide leave the body with each exhalation. Letting your exhale last longer than your inhale lets you oxygenate more efficiently and signals your nervous system to calm.

With your first breath, you might imagine leaving the stress of your workday behind you like discarded armor. With the second, you might release your to-do list into the wind. With the third, you can set a simple, gentle intention. It could be something as simple as, "My intention for this time is to slow down and awaken my senses," or "I intend to be present and receive whatever this place has to offer me today."

Critically, make a conscious decision to silence your phone and, ideally, put it away completely. Airplane mode is your greatest ally on this mission: treat it like a superpower. You are stepping across a threshold into a different world for a little while, a world where your senses, not your thoughts, are your primary guides.

Slow Down Significantly: The Liberating Art of the Unhurried Pace

Once you've mindfully crossed that threshold, begin to walk at a completely unhurried pace. For most of us, so deeply conditioned by the relentless pace of modern life, this is often the most challenging yet ultimately most rewarding part of the entire practice. You must consciously, repeatedly permit yourself to move without a goal. This is significant in our achievement-obsessed world. Release any urge to rush or to achieve a certain distance. Your only destination is the richness of the present moment.

Let your curiosity and your senses guide your movement, imagining how a child would discover something in the natural world for the first time. If a particular patch of moss catches your eye, pause. If a bird's song calls to you, stop and listen. Allow yourself to wander without a plan. When you intentionally slow down your body, you give your senses the time and space they need to truly open up and perceive the world with astonishing depth and clarity.

Phase 3: The Core Practice --Awakening Your Senses with Gentle Invitations

Think of these suggestions not as a rigid checklist, but as gentle, open-ended invitations to explore your environment through different sensory doorways. There's no need to do them all or to follow them in any specific order. Choose the ones that feel most appealing on any given day. Spend several unhurried minutes exploring each chosen invitation. This is where the deep nervous system regulation and mental restoration truly happen-where the magic unfolds.

Invitation: Noticing and Appreciating Motion

Soften your gaze from its usual sharp, analytical focus. Allow your visual awareness to broaden gently like a camera lens opening wide. For the next few minutes, become attuned to all the myriad forms of subtle and overt movement constantly occurring in any living natural setting.

Notice the gentle and almost hypnotic sway of branches and leaves in the breeze, like the Earth breathing. Follow the slow, majestic drift of clouds across the vast canvas of the sky. Track the quick, darting, and often delightfully unpredictable flight of an insect or a bird. Observe the way sunlight shifts and how dappled patterns continuously dance and play across the ground and tree trunks, creating a living, ever-changing mosaic.

Witness all this movement, this constant aliveness, with open, receptive eyes. This practice of observing gentle, non-threatening motion is deeply soothing to our ancient nervous system, signaling safety and peace.

Five-Minute Motion Practice: When time is tight, practice Movement Spotting. Find any outdoor space and spend five minutes identifying different types of motion: obvious ones like cars or people, then subtle ones like grass bending, leaves trembling, or shadows shifting. This rapid visual scanning activates the same attention-restoration mechanisms as longer sessions.

When Your Mind Wanders: During motion observation, anxious thoughts often manifest as a feeling that you're not seeing anything interesting. This is your goal-oriented mind trying to turn the practice into an achievement test. Remind yourself that the goal is simply to look, not to see anything spectacular. Every time you notice judgment arising (This is boring. I'm not good at this), simply return your attention to one specific movement: the edge of a leaf trembling, the pattern of shadows shifting, the way light moves across a surface.

Invitation: Listening Beyond Hearing

Now, shift your primary awareness to your sense of hearing. Prepare to be amazed by what you've been missing. If you feel safe and comfortable, you might gently close your eyes for a few moments. This intentional reduction of visual input can significantly enhance your auditory perception, almost as if you're turning up the volume on the world.

Your ears, bombarded all day by the mechanical hum and sudden jolts of indoor life, can reset in minutes outside. Open your ears wide and listen with the curiosity of a sound detective.

Tune into the full, rich, and layered soundscape of the place you are in. What is the closest sound you can discern now? Maybe it's the whisper of your own breath, the rustle of your clothing, or the soft thud of your own heartbeat.

Now, allow your awareness to expand outward like ripples in a pond. What is the next layer of sound? The dry rustle of fallen leaves as a small creature moves nearby? The more vibrant, almost musical whisper of wind moving through the high canopy of leaves above you? Can you hear the persistent, almost electric hum of insects? The gentle murmur of flowing water, if you're near a stream?

Continue to expand your listening like an audio zoom lens. What is the most distant sound you can detect? Maybe the faint hum of traffic, the call of a bird high overhead, or the distant barking of a dog. As you listen, notice the unique qualities of each sound. Are they sharp or soft? High-pitched or low? Rhythmic or erratic?

Listen more deeply. If you hear nothing, you might notice that even the silence itself has a presence. It lowers heart rate, blood pressure, and cortisol levels. It also lowers activity in the brain's amygdala (aka fear center) and elevates parasympathetic tone. At the same time, the part of your brain that processes sound–your auditory cortex–tunes itself more finely, becomes more sensitive, and subtle sounds stand out more clearly and sharply.

Five-Minute Sound Practice: Practice Sound Spotting. Challenge yourself to identify 10 sounds in five minutes. Start with the obvious, then train your ear to find the subtle. This rapid auditory scanning activates the same attention-restoration mechanisms as longer sessions.

When Your Mind Wanders: When your mind inevitably drifts to your to-do list during the listening practice, don't fight the thoughts like they're the enemy. Instead, use the noting technique: silently thinking when you notice your mind has wandered, then gently guide your attention back to the most prominent sound you can hear right now. Each time you notice and return, you're strengthening your mindfulness muscle. Wandering is not failure; noticing and returning is success.

Invitation: Exploring the Natural Palette

Shift your attention now to the visual. Begin with the color green, the dominant hue of most natural environments. Challenge yourself to see beyond the simple label green. How many shades, tones, and variations of green can you distinguish? The deep emerald of mature oak leaves? The silvery-green of sage? The bright chartreuse of new spring growth? The dark, almost black-green of pine needles?

Move closer to examine textures. Run your eyes along the layered patterns of tree bark. Is it smooth, deeply furrowed, or peeling in distinctive ways? Notice how moss grows in velvet-soft cushions, how lichen creates abstract art on rocks, how fern fronds unfurl in perfect mathematical spirals called fractals.

Look for the interplay of light and shadow, which is nature's own light show. Notice how the quality of light differs between dense shade and an open meadow, and how certain leaves seem to glow when backlit by the sun. This intense visual focus naturally quiets mental chatter because your brain can't simultaneously process detailed visual information and run anxious thought loops.

Invitation: Breathe the Atmosphere

Now turn your attention to your sense of smell, your direct line to ancient memory. Take deep, conscious breaths, drawing the forest air deeply into your lungs like you're sampling fine wine. What do you smell? The earthy, rich scent of decomposing leaves? The clean, sharp smell of pine? The sweet fragrance of wildflowers? The mineral scent of rocks warmed by the sun?

Remember, you are inhaling those immune-boosting tree-aromas, which are part of nature's own pharmacy that has been under research and development for millions of years.

Three-Minute Scent Practice: Practice Scent Sampling. Take 10 deep, conscious breaths in any outdoor space, noticing how each breath smells different from indoor air. Even city air carries traces of earth, plants, and weather. This micro-practice can be done while waiting for a bus, during a work break, or while walking to your car.

Invitation: Cultivating Interconnection

For this final invitation, expand your awareness to the entire living system you're standing within: trees do communicate both underground and in the air.

Beneath your feet, tree roots connect through vast fungal networks: what scientists call the wood wide web. On the roots themselves, mycorrhizal fungi transfer carbon, nutrients, and even chemical signals of stress or support between plants. Oxygen is released from leaves, and carbon dioxide is released when you exhale. Plants, in a direct way, fuel our breathing, and we help to fuel theirs. As you picture these cycles, let yourself feel awe.

You're not a separate observer, you're a participant. You are not separate from this environment; you are part of it. You are engaged in an ancient dance of mutual exchange and reciprocity. You are an inseparable, important part of the living web that sustains us all.

Allow yourself to feel a sense of belonging, of being held and supported by something infinitely larger and more stable than your individual concerns and worries. Reclaiming your health, your vitality, your 7% isn't about getting back to nature. It's about remembering that you are nature.

Integration: Carrying the Forest Home

The integration phase is where the temporary calm of your forest-bathing session biologically shifts into lasting resilience. This is the bridge that carries the nervous system reset into your daily life.

The Physiological Check-In: Before leaving your nature space, spend two to three minutes conducting a gentle body scan like a health detective. Notice what feels different from when you arrived. Has the tension in your shoulders shifted? Is your breathing deeper or slower? Can you feel your heartbeat more clearly? This isn't about judging what you feel. It's about becoming aware of the changes so you can recognize them in the future.

The Sensory Bridge Technique: Select one sensory memory from your session. Perhaps it's the sound of wind in the leaves, the feeling of bark under your palm, or the scent of earth after rain. Practice recalling this sensory anchor vividly. This becomes your portable reset button, accessible anywhere, anytime. Research shows that sensory memories linked to relaxation states can trigger similar nervous system responses when recalled later, even in stressful environments.

Setting Your Carry-Forward Intention: Choose one specific quality from your forest-bathing experience to carry into the next part of your day. It's like selecting the perfect tool for the job ahead. It might be the patience you felt while watching clouds, the stability you experienced leaning against a tree, or the curiosity you discovered while examining moss. Identify this quality clearly and make a conscious intention to embody it in your next interaction or task.

The First-Hour Protocol: The hour immediately following forest bathing is important for maintaining the benefits. Avoid immediately diving into high-stress activities. If you must return to work or family demands, carry the pace with you. Move a little slower, speak a little more softly, and take conscious breaths before responding to requests. You're protecting the nervous system reset you've just achieved.

Nature Notes & Doctor It Up! Your Field Observations

The Paradox of Stillness: Notice how when you first stop moving in nature, your mind actually becomes more agitated before it settles. This is your overstimulated nervous system literally detoxing from its habitual state of hypervigilance. The restlessness you feel isn't a sign you're doing it wrong; it's proof the medicine is working.

The 20-Minute Mark: Pay attention to what happens around the 20-minute mark of your forest-bathing session. This is often when the cortisol washing begins. Your shoulders might spontaneously drop, your breathing naturally deepens, and you might notice you're seeing details that were invisible when you first arrived. This is your nervous system finally downshifting.

The Scent Memory Portal: Observe how certain forest smells can instantly transport you to childhood memories or evoke emotional responses. This is your limbic brain recognizing the ancient chemical signatures of safety and home. These phytoncide compounds are speaking directly to the most primitive parts of your nervous system.

The Sound-Layering Effect: Notice how natural soundscapes have an almost infinite complexity that never becomes annoying, unlike artificial sounds. A city street has maybe 3-5 distinct sound sources, but a forest can have 50 or more, yet they create harmony rather than chaos. This is nature's version of white noise therapy.

The Micro-Movement Medicine: Watch for the tiny movements you miss in regular life: the sometimes imperceptible sway of spider silk, the slow dance of shadows. These micro-movements are calming to our ancient visual processing systems.

The Breath Shift: Track how your breathing pattern changes without conscious effort. Within 10-15 minutes of slow forest walking, most people's respiratory rate drops and their exhales naturally lengthen. The environment is literally teaching your body how to relax.

Doctor It Up!

Amplify the Phytoncide Pharmacy: On days when you need maximum immune support (during cold season, periods of high stress, or when you're feeling run down) seek specific tree species known for their potent phytoncide emissions. Coniferous trees like pine, fir, and cedar are absolute phytoncide powerhouses. Take deliberate, deep breaths near these trees, especially on humid days when the air is thick with these healing compounds.

Engineer Your Perfect HRV Session: To maximize the benefits of heart rate variability, combine your forest bathing with specific breathing techniques. Once you've settled into the environment (around the 15-minute mark), practice *coherent breathing*: inhaling for five counts and exhaling for five counts, creating a six-breath-per-minute rhythm. This specific pattern, combined with the natural environment, creates optimal conditions for parasympathetic activation. You can actually see this in real time with a wearable HRV monitor, and most smartwatches and wearables.

Create Sensory Anchors: Choose one specific sensory experience from each session, like the particular scent of damp moss, the sound of wind in oak leaves, or the texture of a particular tree bark, and consciously anchor it in your memory. Later, when you're stuck in traffic or facing a stressful meeting, you can recall this sensory anchor to trigger an immediate relaxation response.

Optimize Your Circadian Forest Bathing: Time your sessions strategically for maximum benefit. Morning forest bathing (within two hours of sunrise) helps reset your circadian rhythm and provides natural bright light therapy for mood regulation. Evening sessions (two to three hours before sunset) maximize the cortisol-lowering effects as your body naturally prepares for rest.

Weather-Specific Protocols: Don't just endure different weather: find the silver lining. Light rain amplifies the release of petrichor (that distinctive earth after rain smell) and negative ions, both of which have mood-lifting properties. Fresh snow creates an almost supernatural quiet that can induce powerful meditative states. Fog and mist provide natural aromatherapy as they carry concentrated plant essences. Overcast days often make colors more saturated and sound more distinct.

Your Outdoor Rx Action Space

My Forest-Bathing Prescription:

Location Scout: My chosen sanctuary is:
_____

Time Commitment: I will practice for _____ minutes, _____ times per week

Best Times for My Schedule: _____

My Backup Urban Spots (for when my primary location isn't accessible):
_____

My Sensory Preferences (which invitations resonate most):
☐ Motion observation ☐ Deep listening ☐ Visual exploration
☐ Scent awareness ☐ Touch and texture ☐ Interconnection awareness

My Personal Barriers and Solutions:

Barrier:_____
Solution:_____
Barrier:_____
Solution: _____

Week 1 Commitment: I will forest bathe on these specific days/times:
Day 1:_____
Day 2:_____
Day 3: _____

My Integration Ritual: After each session, I will
_____

Progress Tracking: I'll measure my success by noticing changes in: ☐ Sleep quality ☐ Stress response ☐ Mood stability ☐ Attention span ☐ Physical tension ☐ Other: _____

Emergency Forest-Bathing Plan (for high-stress days): When I feel overwhelmed, I will spend _____ minutes at _____ focusing on _____

My Accountability Partner: _____ will support my practice by _____.

Sensory Anchor Collection: I will build a library of calming sensory memories:
Sight: _____
Sound: _____
Smell: _____
Touch: _____
Movement: _____

Urban Practice Notes: When I can't access my primary sanctuary, I will: ☐ Practice window forest bathing for _____ minutes ☐ Visit my backup single-tree spot ☐ Use my pocket park protocol ☐ Focus on _____

Weather Adaptation Plan:

Rainy days: _____
Snowy conditions: _____
Windy weather: _____
Overcast skies: _____

Micro-Dose Schedule (for busy days):

3-minute breathing practice: _____
5-minute motion observation: _____
10-minute full sensory sampling: _____

Chapter 4: Move Like You Mean It

Introduction: The Mission to Create Mindful Movement Outdoors

This chapter is about reclaiming something you already know how to do: move. But not as punishment or to hit a step count, or because an app reminded you to do so. Here, we view outdoor movement as medicine and examine the proven health benefits of physical activity in nature.

You'll see how even modest activity like walking, stretching, and gardening becomes more restorative when it happens near trees, beside water, or under the sky.

> **Watercooler Fact:**
> Green Exercise Advantage: People report 20% lower perceived exertion when exercising outdoors versus indoors at the same intensity.

Personal records and rep counts have a place in strength and fitness. But movement outside doesn't try to hit either. Instead, green exercise suggests shifting your relationship to movement entirely when outside. Green Exercise is about experiencing and moving outdoors rather than sweating.

When you're outside, moving through real terrain rather than staring at a treadmill screen, your body responds with greater efficiency, and your mind with greater clarity. And your long-term, outside-the-gym blood pressure actually drops more with green exercise than indoor work. So you're not just getting your heart rate up. You're lowering cortisol, improving immune function, enhancing neuroplasticity (see Glossary) and increasing both healthspan and longevity.

Walking on uneven, natural terrain requires 28 percent more energy than walking on a treadmill or flat pavement. That extra demand recruits stabilizing muscles, strengthens joints, and improves balance. It also produces a greater cardiovascular load at the same perceived effort, meaning you get a greater metabolic return without feeling like you are working harder. A 30-minute walk on a woodland path offers a far greater return than 30 minutes on a suburban sidewalk.

Regular green exercise of 150-300 minutes a week reduces mortality risk by nearly a quarter, making it one of the most powerful low-cost longevity tools we have. You'll also see that Green Exercise delivers a double serving of nutritional benefits.

First, outdoor movement exposes skin to UVB rays, triggering natural Vitamin D production—as you know, important for strong bones, telomere protection, and a resilient immune system.

Second, outdoor exercise itself delivers unique metabolic and cognitive benefits that indoor training cannot replicate, from a more even-mood to greater insulin sensitivity. Adding the outdoors to your indoor workout or shifting your whole workout outdoors doesn't just build muscle, balance and flexibility; it amplifies every healthy choice you make at the table.

Indoor Epidemic

This chapter offers a menu of nature-based movement options that can fit any body, lifestyle, or ability. The science is clear: after age 50, we naturally lose 1–2% of muscle mass, strength, and power each year unless we actively train against it. The real master keys to maintaining independence into later life are resistance work to preserve muscle power and balance, and gait training to prevent falls.

Practicing resistance and balance exercises outdoors offers unique advantages. Sunlight entrains your circadian rhythm, natural surfaces challenge your stability in ways a flat gym floor never can, and green environments lower stress hormones while enhancing focus. A skilled trainer can help you with consistency and form, but even without a trainer, working out outside can be practiced safely and effectively.

> **Watercooler Fact:**
> The average cost for an hour of a skilled personal trainer's time is **$55 per hour**, though the price typically ranges from **$40 to $100**.

Whether it's a sunrise stretch on the beach, a walk after dinner through your neighborhood, or a more vigorous hike, the key to continuing to move for longevity is finding what feels good and returning to it often. Because when movement is tied to pleasure, place, and purpose, it becomes a habit worth keeping.

If your child is dependent on screens, the answer is rarely more rules. The answer is better choices. Children lack the neurological maturity to resist devices engineered for constant stimulation. What they need is access to real-life experiences that compete with the digital pull. The outdoors is not a wellness option. It is a developmental requirement.

Activities like movement, art, music, and growing food return a child to presence and sensory engagement. These are the experiences that restore attention and emotional steadiness. They provide the satisfaction that screens promise but never deliver. Parents can create a culture at home where time away from devices is expected and protected. When that happens, children discover what it feels like to be fully alive again.

When movement habits are rooted in nature, it's not just green exercise. It's a potent upgrade for your entire being.

The Why: Why Moving Outdoors Isn't Just Exercise, It's a Potent Upgrade for Your Entire Being

I write exercise prescriptions for patients and here's the upgrade: Green Exercise. It frees you from the indoor cage, letting you breathe fresh air and let in natural light to recharge your body and sharpen your mind.

Regular physical activity in natural settings has been shown to reduce cardiovascular risk, including a 9% lower likelihood of developing high blood pressure. And the environment itself matters: people who live in greener areas usually have longer telomeres, mentioned earlier, which are the protective caps on DNA that serve as a marker of cellular aging. Nature exposure may directly slow biological aging, not just indirectly.

> **Watercooler Fact:**
> Telomere Protection: People living in greener areas have longer telomeres, a key biomarker of slower cellular aging.

For older adults, the impact is especially striking. Leisure-time physical activity, often done outdoors, is linked with a 16% reduction in all-cause mortality, even in those without so-called longevity genes.

The difference between merely being outside and moving outside with intention is biological. Incidental outdoor exposure delivers light and air, but it does not load the system as much as green exercise does. A brisk walk on a tree-lined trail is not just exercise in a prettier setting. It is a different biological signal.

Active vs. Passive Exposure

Passive exposure matters. A patient recovering from surgery in a room with a window view of trees needs fewer pain medications and heals faster than a patient staring through a window at a brick wall. But the gains multiply when you move. Movement outdoors layers physical activity on top of sensory immersion, producing additive benefits for stress, mood, metabolism, and immunity.

This is why green exercise consistently outperforms the same workout done indoors. A treadmill in a gym lowers blood pressure. A trail walk lowers blood pressure and cortisol simultaneously, while enhancing working memory and mood.

Urban Nature, Same Power

The excuse of not having wilderness nearby does not justify not exercising outside. Urban parks provide 80–90 percent of the benefits of wild nature. Even green spaces with 20–30 percent vegetation coverage deliver measurable reductions in depression and anxiety. Walking loops in a city park, cycling on a riverside path, or practicing yoga in a backyard with trees all count as green exercise. The body responds to cues from greenery, the sky, and natural sounds.

Your Prescription

Every incidental minute outdoors is an opportunity waiting to be converted. Every walk to your car in the parking lot could be a walk around the block under trees. Every lunch break to the downtown sandwich shop could be a brisk circuit in a park. Those two hours push you over the 120-minute line where survival curves shift, and they begin building toward the 200–300 minute plateau where longevity gains peak.

The efficiency is staggering: two hours of deliberate green movement per week is one of the lowest cost, highest return interventions available in medicine.

Among the elderly, just 15 minutes of walking several times a week has been associated with a 40% lower risk of death. That's a meaningful extension in functional, independent life.

What also sets outdoor movement apart from its indoor counterpart is how it feels. People consistently report higher energy and lower perceived exertion when exercising outside, even when the physical workload is the same. The novelty and complexity of natural settings may also stimulate greater increases in brain-derived neurotrophic factor (BDNF), which supports learning, memory, and mood. Green Exercise isn't just good for your body: it helps your mind stay sharper, longer.

Let's begin this mission with a fundamental truth: you already know that exercise is medicine. The evidence is overwhelming. If exercise could be bottled and sold as a pill, it would be the most valuable and widely prescribed pharmaceutical on the planet.

But here's the secret, the revolutionary insight that this chapter is built on: where you take this medicine matters just as much as that you take it. The environment in which you choose to move your body is not merely a passive backdrop; it is an active ingredient in the prescription. It can either dilute the medicine or it can amplify its effects exponentially.

Engaging in physical activity in natural environments offers a multiplier effect. It combines the well-established physiological and psychological benefits of moving your body with the incredible restorative, dynamic, and multi-sensory healing qualities of the natural world. Here are five ways movement rebuilds your brain, beats stress, and rewires your biology.

1. The Science of Mood and Mind: A Direct Counteroffensive on Stress, Cortisol, and Anxiety

This is where Green Exercise truly shines and where you will probably feel the most immediate and measurable benefits. For anyone battling the chronic stress, persistent anxiety, or low-grade blahs that are the hallmarks of modern indoor life, this is your most accessible and potent prescription.

The Double Dose of Calm: Dual Benefits

When you exercise, your body releases endorphins, the brain's natural mood-elevating and pain-relieving chemicals. This is the runner's high, leaving you feeling clear-headed and less stressed after a good workout. When you immerse yourself in a natural environment, as we learned in the previous chapter, your nervous system receives a powerful signal to relax, reducing stress hormones and shifting you into a state of calm.

Green Exercise combines these two powerful effects into a single, dual benefit dose of well-being. It is a true two-for-one therapy for your mind. Movement plus nature is a powerful combination: the body's calming signal lowers cortisol and anxiety while activity clears tension. That is the physiology of calm.

Studies comparing indoor versus outdoor exercise consistently show that activity in natural settings leads to greater reductions in perceived stress, tension, anxiety, and anger than in urban settings.

A Direct Hit on Your Stress Hormones

Let's talk specifics. Your body's primary activity hormone is cortisol. In the 93% of your day spent indoors, cortisol can spike high and stay high. As we explored in Chapter 3, while necessary in small bursts, chronic cortisol elevation caused by the relentless pressures of modern life is deeply damaging, disrupting sleep, fogging your thinking, promoting fat storage, and contributing to long-term disease risk.

Multiple studies have now confirmed that exposure to green space is directly linked to lower physiological stress, including measurable reductions in salivary cortisol levels.

One of the most cited findings in this field is that a nature exposure of 20-30 minutes can reduce cortisol levels by about 21%. When you combine that calming effect with the stress-reducing power of exercise itself, you create one of the most effective protocols available for resetting your entire stress-response system.

For patients experiencing chronic stress and emotional exhaustion, I often recommend a 30-minute walk in a nearby green space as a first-line intervention. The physiological and psychological benefits of light to moderate activity in natural environments are both immediate and measurable.

A Natural Antidote to Anxiety and Low Mood

The data on Green Exercise as a tool for mental health is incredibly encouraging. Large-scale population studies have revealed a strong link between access to nature and better mental well-being. One study found that urban populations who engage in regular visits to outdoor green spaces for just 30 minutes or more per week were associated with a 7% lower prevalence of depression. Another compelling finding is that greater access to green space is associated with lower antidepressant prescription rates by up to 9%.

Side-by-side trials show that exercising in nature boosts mood and calms anxiety more than doing the same routine indoors. This is because you are not just moving your body; you are simultaneously immersing your senses in a rich, restorative environment. The combination has a measurablely calming and uplifting effect on your nervous system and your emotional state.

The Revitalization Factor: More Than Just Energy

One of the most consistent findings in the research is that, compared to slogging it out indoors, Green Exercise is strongly associated with greater feelings of revitalization, more positive engagement, and a greater surge in energy. This is a feeling many of us have intuitively. The walk in the park on your lunch break leaves you feeling refreshed and alive in a way that a session on a stationary bike under fluorescent lights rarely does.

As a trained chef, I know that fresh, vibrant ingredients are what make a dish; fresh air, dynamic light, and natural scenery are the essential ingredients that make your movement meal truly come alive.

2. The Cognitive Upgrade: Reclaiming Your Focus and Fueling Your Brain

As we explored in the previous chapter, our capacity for 'directed attention', the kind of focused, top-down concentration required for demanding work, is a limited resource that becomes easily fatigued by the demands of our screen-saturated lives. As we found out with Forest Bathing, Attention Restoration Theory (ART) (see Glossary) proposes that natural environments are uniquely suited to restoring this depleted cognitive resource. Again, they allow for 'soft fascination' that captures our attention effortlessly, allowing our overtaxed directed-attention networks to take a much-needed break, to rest, and to recharge.

> **Watercooler Fact:**
>
> **CO_2 Cognitive Drain:** Indoor carbon dioxide levels above 1,000 ppm can reduce decision-making and cognitive performance by 15%.

When you combine this restorative environment with physical movement, the effects are amplified. The rhythmic nature of walking or running can help to quiet the brain's Narrator of me while the natural scenery provides the soft fascination needed to recharge your focus. This is why so many people report that their best ideas come to them while walking outdoors.

The data backs this up. A University of Michigan study found that a walk in a park but not an urban walk improves short-term memory. In a test of repeating random number strings forward and backward, scores rose about 20% versus a same-length walk on a busy city street. The park walk restored the mental bandwidth needed for focus and working memory.

You can test this yourself with the same test psychologists use:

Start with these: Forward: 7—1—9—4—6; Backward: 3—8—2—5—9.

Now take a 10–15-minute walk in a park or along a tree-lined street.

When you return, test yourself again with a new set of numbers: Forward: 4—9—6—2—7; Backward: 8—5—1—7—3.

Using a fresh set of numbers is an advantage because you're not just repeating from memory, but instead measuring how much sharper and more flexible your brain has become. The backward set might feel easier after your walk, because your brain's executive function has been rebooted and refreshed by nature.

BDNF: The Brain's Best Friend

Exercise is one of the most potent ways to stimulate the production of a remarkable protein called Brain-Derived Neurotrophic Factor (BDNF). Think of BDNF as Miracle-Gro or fertilizer for your brain. This remarkable protein both feeds neurons and grows new ones, rewiring your brain for sharper focus, stronger memory, and greater resilience. Healthy BDNF levels are vital for a sharp, resilient, and plastic brain.

Unlike the delays and sometime monotony of indoor exercise, working out in complex, stimulating natural environments may boost BDNF production more effectively. Your brain's constant need to process new information, navigate changing terrain, and respond to dynamic surroundings provides additional stimulus for releasing this critical molecule.

The possibility that Green Exercise provides a superior boost to your brain's own fertilizer is a compelling reason to take your workout to the trails.

3. The Cardiovascular and Metabolic Perks: Your Physical Health

While the mental benefits of Green Exercise are often felt most immediately, the advantages for your long-term physical health are measurable and well documented. This is where the practice becomes a powerful form of preventive medicine, directly combating the metabolic and cardiovascular damage caused by the Indoor Epidemic.

An Unexpected Tool for Longevity

Green exercise offers a survival advantage that the gym alone cannot. A 2026 analysis of over 111000 people followed for 34 years published in *BMJ Medicine* found that participating in a wide range of physical activities lowered all-cause mortality by 19%. That benefit was independent of total amount of exercise. Walking was the top exercise for pure survival, reducing mortality risk by 17%. Digging and chopping protected against a respiratory-related death, more than any other exercise.

Living in a greener neighborhood improves your blood pressure and also lowers your risk of heart disease. The Louisville Green Heart Project, backed by grants from the NIH and the Nature Conservancy, showed that people living in the newly green area of town reduced their inflammation levels by up to 20% in just a few years. The blood test that was measured, hsCRP, is an even stronger indicator of heart attack risk than cholesterol levels!

A Powerful Tool Against Type 2-Diabetes

The Indoor Epidemic is often accompanied by a sedentary lifestyle, which is a primary driver of metabolic dysfunction. A lack of physical activity impairs your body's ability to manage blood sugar, leading to insulin resistance and, eventually, Type 2 diabetes.

Green Exercise is a direct and potent countermeasure to developing diabetes. Make your 7% count with not just a look out the window, but by moving outside to feel the breeze on your skin.

It's also well known that more green space exposure means less Type 2 Diabetes. The mechanisms are twofold. First, being outside encourages more overall physical activity. Second, being outside seems to affect blood sugar regulation. A stunning study on diabetic patients found that a 30-minute walk in a forest lowered their post-meal blood sugar by an average of 40 mg/dL. This shows a powerful, immediate metabolic benefit that can help manage existing diabetes and prevent its onset.

The Sunshine Vitamin: A Crucial Co-Benefit

One of the most unavoidable consequences of an indoor life is Vitamin D deficiency, unless actively and consistently supplemented. Moving your body outdoors, especially when the sun is higher in the sky (mid-morning to mid-afternoon, depending on the season and your latitude), provides your skin with the opportunity to synthesize Vitamin D from sunlight's UVB rays.

Vitamin D is mandatory for bone health (preventing osteoporosis), robust immune function, and mood regulation. It is important to always practice safe sun exposure. Being mindful of the UV index, your skin type, and avoiding sunburn at all costs is just smart. But the opportunity to naturally produce this critical hormone is a significant added benefit of taking your workout outdoors.

4. The Stick-With-It Factor: The Psychology of Sustainable Movement

This might be the most important section. From a clinical perspective, the most effective exercise program on the planet is useless if you don't actually do it consistently. The biggest challenge for most people is not knowing what to do, but finding the motivation and enjoyment to keep doing it. This is where Green Exercise reveals its secret weapon: adherence.

It Actually Feels Easier

Here's a fascinating "a-ha!" moment for anyone who has ever dreaded a workout. Several studies and meta-analyses have found that people consistently report a lower rate of perceived exertion (RPE) after engaging in Green Exercise compared to performing the exact same workout indoors.

So, a 30-minute run on a forest trail might feel easier and more pleasant than a 30-minute run on a treadmill, even if your heart rate and calorie burn are the same. The engaging natural scenery seems to act as a positive distraction from the feelings of physical effort and fatigue. This lower RPE can allow you to potentially go longer, push harder, or, most importantly, simply enjoy the experience more.

Movement for Longevity

Movement is the best drug to prevent premature aging, and the emphasis should evolve as we do. In your 30s, aerobic and strength training dominate. By your 40s and 50s, progressive resistance training (PRT) becomes just as important.

After 60, the hierarchy is clear: power and resistance first, balance and gait second, aerobic third. Nature is the ideal environment for this work. Carrying loads in the garden or climbing a hill challenges strength and power, while walking trails with their roots and slopes continuously trains balance and stability. These movements prepare you not just for exercise, but for the demands of real life.

The reasoning is simple and clinical. After midlife, the greatest threat to independence isn't hypertension or diabetes: it's falls. Roughly one in three older adults experiences a fall each year, often with lasting consequences. That's why experts recommend PRT on 2–3 non-consecutive days per week at 70–85% of maximum effort, along with balance and gait training at least three days per week, which can reduce fall risk by up to 40%. Nature amplifies both: a lunge on soft ground demands stabilization no gym floor requires, and a push-up on a log recruits more core and balance than an exercise machine. Outdoors, the environment becomes a training partner in resilience.

The Joy Factor: Maximizing Your What's In It For Me? (WIFM)

Behavioral science is crystal clear on this point: intrinsic enjoyment is one of the most potent predictors of long-term adherence to any health habit. By tapping into the mood-boosting, stress-reducing, and aesthetically pleasing qualities of nature, Green Exercise dramatically increases the joy factor of physical activity. This skyrockets the probability that you will make it a regular, valued, and definitive part of your life.

If you've struggled for years to stay consistent with an exercise program, the missing ingredient might not be more willpower; it might be a dose of nature.

Building Real-World Functional Fitness

Finally, moving your body in nature builds a more resilient and capable body. Activities common in Green Exercise, like hiking or trail running, involve constantly navigating varied and uneven terrain and are fantastic for your body.

Green Exercise gently challenges your balance, sharpens your proprioception (your body's sixth sense of its position in space), and builds functional strength in the small stabilizing muscles around your ankles, knees, hips, and core. The flat, predictable surfaces of a gym can't compete: it's fitness that translates directly to navigating the real world with more confidence, grace, and a reduced risk of injury.

5. The Emerging Frontiers: Your Gut and Your Genes

Two of the most exciting new frontiers involve its potential impact on our gut microbiome (see Glossary) and even the aging process at a cellular level.

There is a fascinating and emerging hypothesis that exercising in natural environments provides a powerful double benefit for your gut microbes. We know that exercise itself can positively influence the diversity and composition of your gut microbiome. We also know that being outdoors exposes you to a much greater diversity of environmental microbes from the soil, the air, and plants.

Green Exercise likely creates a dual benefit, modulating your internal ecosystem through both movement and microbial exchanges with the environment. A healthier, more diverse gut microbiome could be another pathway through which Green Exercise improves stress response, mood, and overall neurological health. They're all critical for healthy aging and longevity.

Living Greener, Living Longer? The Telomere Connection

This is perhaps the most tantalizing area of research. Several large-scale epidemiological studies have found a significant association between people living in areas with more residential green space and reduced all-cause mortality. They tend to live longer, with specific reductions noted for cardiovascular and respiratory mortality.

Even more intriguingly, some research has suggested that individuals living in greener areas have been observed to have longer telomere lengths. The reduced chronic physiological stress, lower systemic inflammation, and decreased oxidative stress facilitated by nature exposure are known to help protect telomere length. The landscapes around us may be quietly scripting the pace of our cellular aging and shaping longevity at the level of our DNA.

The How-To (Your Mission): Move Like You Mean It

Your energizing mission, should you choose to embrace this pathway to greater vitality, is to engage consciously and consistently in some form of enjoyable, personally meaningful, and sustainable outdoor movement for approximately 15 to 45 minutes (or even longer, if it feels fantastic and your schedule allows) on most days of the week.

The critical shift here, the real game-changer that will determine your long-term success, is not to focus on the numbers.

Instead, just try to appreciate the positive feeling of being physically active. Your goal is to build a mindful and appreciative connection with your physical self and your natural surroundings, and to finish your session feeling better than when you started: energized, refreshed, mentally clearer, and maybe even a little more joyful and alive.

Forget the 'no pain, no gain' meme that's left so many of us burned out or injured. Your body isn't a machine to hack; it's a sensing, responsive vessel that only runs sustainably on joyful, purposeful movement. Not will or force.

When you treat activity as self-care instead of self-discipline, it stops feeling like a chore. You sometimes look forward to it and want to start it. Movement actually becomes a source of energy, like your breath, not something that drains it.

Your Menu of Joyful Movement: An Invitation to Explore

Try joining a local walking group, sports club, or weekend hike. These activities try to connect, not compete. You're connecting, not just with others, but with how to use your breath, and with the ability and consciousness of moving without metrics. Leave your phone in your bag, and you might just rediscover the pleasure of shared effort and old-fashioned fun.

This is how joyful movement becomes more than exercise: it becomes a small rebellion against optimization culture. We are throwing out the rulebook that says a workout must involve a gym, a punishing routine, or a feeling of dread.

Think of this next section as a menu: many options designed to nourish your body and mind. You're not expected to sample everything. Just notice what stirs your curiosity, what feels doable, even fun. The best exercise on paper is useless if you don't actually do it.

The Foundational Superstar: Walking

What It Is: Walking is the most underrated, accessible, and versatile form of Green Exercise on the planet. It is the cornerstone of a sustainable outdoor movement practice.

> **Watercooler Fact**
>
> **Shoe Contamination:** Nearly all outdoor shoes carry fecal bacteria, carcinogenic toxins from asphalt, and synthetic pesticides indoors.

Who It's For: This is for everyone. It is the perfect entry point for someone who has been sedentary for years, as it is low impact and easily scalable. It is an important tool for the high-performance athlete as a form of active recovery. It is for the busy professional who needs to clear their head, the new parent pushing a stroller, and the older adult looking to maintain mobility and cardiovascular health.

Your Mission & Creative Examples:

The Brisk Power Walk: This is your go-to for cardiovascular health. The goal is to walk at a pace that elevates your heart rate and makes you breathe a little harder, yet still allows you to hold a conversation. This type of walking is fantastic for improving insulin sensitivity, burning calories, and boosting your mood through the release of endorphins. Try finding a 1-2-mile loop in a local park and timing yourself, aiming to lower your time over a period of weeks.

The Slow, Mindful Meander: This is about connecting, not conquering. As we explored in the previous chapter, a slow, meandering walk is the foundation of Forest Bathing. On days when you feel stressed, overwhelmed, or mentally fatigued, this is your prescription. Leave the headphones at home. Walk at a snail's pace. Turn your phone to airplane mode. Let your senses guide you instead of your screen. As you walk, notice the breeze on your face, the light shifting through leaves, the small sounds that rarely surface indoors. The experience becomes more than a walk. It becomes a way of remembering what real presence feels like.

This simple act of disconnection is not just a habit: it's a practice of reclaiming attention from a world that wants to monetize it. Your goal is to engage all your senses. Notice the light, the sounds, the smells. This type of walk is less about cardiovascular fitness and more about nervous system regulation and mental restoration.

Move Like You Mean It

Invigorating Interval Walking: This is a brilliant way to boost your metabolism and strengthen your heart efficiently. The concept is simple: alternate periods of faster, more intense walking with periods of slower, recovery-paced walking. For example, you could walk at a moderate pace for 3 minutes, then walk as fast as you can (a power walk, not a run) for 20 seconds. Repeat this cycle 5-8 times. This is a highly effective workout that can be done in just 20-30 minutes.

Watercooler Fact

11-Minute Longevity Boost: Just 11 minutes of daily outdoor activity lowers risk of premature death by 23%, across nearly 200 studies.

The Social Stroll: Combine the benefits of movement with the power of human connection (the focus of our next chapter). Schedule a regular walk-and-talk with a friend, your partner, or a family member. Conversations often flow more easily and authentically when walking side by side in a relaxed outdoor setting rather than sitting face to face in a noisy cafe. If 86% of your life is walled in, and 7% is in vehicles, let part of your 7% be your longevity goal.

Playful Walking Variations: Challenge your brain and body by breaking out of your normal walking pattern. Try walking backward for short stretches (20-30 steps) on a safe, clear, and perfectly flat path. This is challenging and fantastic for improving your balance and coordination. You can also try carioca (grapevine steps) or side-shuffling to engage different muscles in your hips and legs.

Nature's Yoga Studio: Stretching, Mobility & Mindful Flow

What It Is: This is about taking practices that cultivate a deep mind-body connection such as yoga, Tai Chi, Qigong, and mobility work and moving them from the confines of an indoor studio into the expansive, sensory-rich environment of the outdoors.

Who It's For: This practice is a powerful antidote for anyone who feels stiff, tight, and disconnected from their body due to long hours of sitting. It is for the person seeking to improve flexibility, release tension, and cultivate a sense of inner calm and grace. It is also for the athlete or active individual who knows the importance of recovery and mobility for injury prevention.

Your Mission & Creative Examples:

Sunrise Salutations: Pro tip: face the actual rising sun. Find a quiet spot in a park or your backyard as the day begins. Feel the warmth of the early light on your skin as you move through the poses. This practice powerfully combines the benefits of movement with the circadian-setting power of morning light from Chapter 1.

Tai Chi Under the Trees: The slow, gentle, flowing movements of Tai Chi or Qigong are perfectly suited to an outdoor setting. Practicing under the canopy of a large, mature tree can create a sense of steadiness and peace. The fresh air and natural surroundings amplify the focus on slow, deliberate movement and coordinated breathing.

Dynamic Mobility Breaks: You don't need a full hour. Take a 10-minute mobility snack in your backyard during a work break. Perform a simple sequence of dynamic, full-body movements: walking lunges with a torso twist, standing cat-cow movements to mobilize your spine, and big arm circles to open up your shoulders. This can be a powerful way to break up long periods of sitting and reenergize your body and mind.

Nature's Obstacle Course: Balance, Agility & Proprioception

What It Is: This is about consciously seeking out and engaging with the varied and uneven terrain of the natural world to train your body's sixth sense, proprioception. Proprioception is your body's innate awareness of its position in space, a constant feedback loop between your brain and your muscles and joints.

A sharp proprioceptive sense is important for good balance, agility, and preventing falls.

Who It's For: This is for everyone, but it is especially critical as we age. It's for the trail runner who wants to navigate technical terrain with more confidence, the older adult who wants to reduce their risk of a debilitating fall, and anyone who wants to build the kind of real-world, functional strength that makes them more resilient in all of life's activities.

Your Mission & Creative Examples:

Walk the Line: Find a stable, low-to-the-ground fallen log (always meticulously check its stability first!), a low, wide curb, or even the clearly defined edge of a garden bed. Carefully and mindfully walk along it, as if on a balance beam. Feel the thousands of micro-adjustments your feet, ankles, and core must make to keep you stable.

Single-Leg Stands: Practice standing on one leg on slightly uneven ground, like a patch of grass or soft dirt. This is significantly more challenging for your stabilizing muscles than standing on a perfectly flat indoor floor. Try to hold for 30 seconds on each leg. To increase the challenge, try closing your eyes for a few seconds.

Playful Agility Drills: Incorporate light, playful agility movements into your walks. Hop from one flat stone to another across a small stream. Practice quick side-shuffles for 10-15 yards. Lightly hop over small, safe obstacles like twigs or low mounds of earth. This retrains your nervous system to be quick and responsive.

Embrace the Trail: The best way to improve your proprioception is to walk or hike regularly on natural, uneven trails. The constant need to adapt to rocks, roots, and changing slopes is the ultimate training for your neuromuscular system.

Recapturing Joy: The Medicine of Play

What It Is: When was the last time you truly allowed yourself to play with uninhibited enthusiasm? For many adults, especially high-achievers and people pleasers, play feels frivolous, unproductive, or even embarrassing. This is a tragic loss. Play is not the opposite of work; it is an important form of restoration. It is a biological necessity for creativity, stress relief, and social bonding. For a true mental escape and stress relief, try an offline analog game—horseshoes or cornhole outside, gin rummy or bridge inside, dominoes or chess inside or outside: they're all easy to play, and hard to master.

Who It's For: This is for anyone who has ever felt drained by endless responsibilities or trapped in a cycle of being always on. Whether you're a burned-out worker, an overwhelmed caregiver, a serious student, or just someone who hasn't laughed out loud at a game for far too long, you need to play. Any adult who has been told that their value lies only in their productivity needs to play again: the fun, connection, and challenge are just as important to the good life, if not more.

Your Mission & Creative Examples:

Toss a Frisbee: There is something primally satisfying about throwing and catching a Frisbee in a wide-open park. It is a simple, joyful activity that gets you moving, laughing, and connecting with a partner.

Fly a Kite: On a breezy afternoon, flying a kite is a beautiful, almost meditative form of play. It connects you directly to the invisible power of the wind and draws your gaze upward to the expansive sky.

Dance Like Nobody's Watching: Put on your favorite upbeat music through your headphones. Find a secluded spot in a park, on a beach, or in your own backyard where you feel uninhibited, and just dance. Move your body however it feels good. This is a powerful, expressive release of stored tension and an act of joyful embodiment.

Play Informal Games: Get a group of friends or family together for a low-stakes game of pickleball, badminton, volleyball, or even bocce ball or horseshoes in the park. The gentle competition, laughter, and shared goal make for a wonderfully connective experience.

Nature Work: The Power of Functional Fitness

What It Is: This is about discovering the significant and comprehensive physical benefits of engaging in purposeful, nature-based tasks. This is fitness that doesn't feel like exercise because it has a tangible, satisfying outcome.

Who It's For: This is perfect for the person who hates formal workouts but loves to be productive and see the results of their hard work. It is for homeowners, gardeners, and anyone who enjoys hands-on projects.

Your Mission & Creative Examples:

Gardening: As we will explore in depth in Chapter 6, gardening is a fantastic full-body workout. Digging strengthens your arms and back, squatting and weeding build leg strength and mobility, and carrying soil and water build core stability.

Mindful Yard Work: When you rake leaves in the autumn, do it vigorously, engaging your core and obliques. When you shovel snow in the winter, treat it like a session of interval training, being mindful to use proper form (bend your knees, keep your back straight) to avoid injury. When you push a manual lawnmower, feel the engagement of your legs and chest.

Community Volunteer Projects: Join a local park cleanup or a trail maintenance day. Hauling bags of trash, clearing brush, or helping to build a new path can be incredibly rewarding work that builds both community and functional strength.

> **Watercooler Fact:**
> **Food Chain Crisis:** One in every three bites of food depends on bee pollination. Yet we're systematically destroying the outdoor spaces they need to survive.

Foraging: Eating in the wild can be wild (never eat mushrooms you find), but foraging can be great exercise and a lot of fun. With proper guidance from a local expert who knows the territory and about food safety, find available berries or edible greens (check out fallingfruit.org for a map) and change your walk into a treasure hunt.

Nature's Gym: Bodyweight Basics with Natural Equipment

What It Is: This is a creative, resourceful, and completely free approach to strength training. It involves seeing the natural and built environment around you as your personal, ever-changing outdoor gym.

Who It's For: Anyone looking for an accessible way to build strength without a gym membership. It is for the person who enjoys creativity and adaptability in their workouts.

Your Mission & Creative Examples:

The Park Bench Station: A sturdy park bench is a versatile piece of workout equipment.

Incline Push-ups: Place your hands on the seat or the back of the bench. The higher your hands are off the ground, the easier the push-up will be. This is a great way to build up to full push-ups.

Triceps Dips: Sit on the edge of the bench, place your hands next to your hips, and slide your body forward. Lower and raise your body by bending your elbows.

Bulgarian Split Squats: Stand a few feet in front of the bench and place the top of your back foot on the seat. Lower your body into a lunge. This is a fantastic exercise for leg strength and stability.

The Tree Anchor: A strong, mature tree can provide excellent support.

Assisted Squats: Face the tree and hold on to the trunk for balance as you perform deep squats, ensuring your form is correct.

Rows with Resistance Bands: Loop a resistance band around the trunk of a sturdy tree and perform rows to strengthen your back muscles.

Tree Sits: Fundamentally a wall sit, but using the solid, grounding presence of a tree for back support.

The Hill Circuit: Natural inclines offer fantastic built-in resistance.

Hill Sprints: Find a moderately steep hill and perform short, all-out sprints, walking back down to recover. This is a powerful high-intensity interval workout.

Walking Lunges: Performing walking lunges up a hill dramatically increases the challenge for your glutes and quads.

The Found Object: Large, stable rocks or securely positioned fallen logs can be used for careful lifting and carrying (simulating farmers' walks), precise step-overs, or even box jumps (always ensure absolute stability first).

By seeing the world through this lens, you realize you are never without a place to build your strength and resilience.

Helpful Tips and Bonus Info (Nature Notes & Doctor It Up!)

You have your mission: to find joy and vitality in outdoor motion. You have the menu of options, your personal invitation to explore what makes your body and spirit come alive. I want to provide you with the advanced training manual. This section is your field guide for making your Green Exercise practice not just something you do, but a deeply rewarding, sustainable, and integrated part of your life.

Here, we will cover the vital principles that modify movement from a task into a powerful form of self-care and medicine. We will discuss how to listen to your body to prevent injury, how to make your practice social and fun, and how to stack your Outdoor Rx doses for a potent, dual benefit. These are the strategies that will ensure your success on this important mission.

Here's the real magic: the true beauty of the Outdoor Rx system isn't just the individual steps; it's how they work together, creating greater effects than the sum of their parts. This isn't about adding more to your plate; it's about maximizing the impact of every single intentional minute you spend outside. This powerful repurposing of time you already spend outside is precisely what supercharges your healthspan and longevity.

Doctor It Up #1: Listen Fiercely to Your Body-- The Golden Rule of Sustainable Movement

This is the most important principle in this entire chapter. Focusing on safety and learning to listen to the subtle (and not-so-subtle) signals of your body is not a sign of weakness. It is the highest form of wisdom in any physical practice. The goal is long-term vitality, not short-term gains at the cost of injury.

The Difference Between Work and Pain: It is critical and important to learn the difference between the healthy sensation of muscle fatigue, like the satisfying burn that signals you are building strength and the sharp, persistent or radiating pain that signals a potential injury.

Healthy exertion feels like a global fatigue in the muscle belly. Warning-sign pain is often localized to a joint, sharp, stabbing, or worsens with movement. Do not push through this kind of pain.

The Art of Gradual Progression: If you are new to exercise or returning after a long break, the principle of gradual progression is your best friend. Start slowly. Increase the intensity, duration, or frequency of your workouts by no more than about 10% per week. This gives your muscles, tendons, and cardiovascular system time to adapt and grow stronger, dramatically reducing your risk of injury.

The Mandatory Warm-Up and Cool-Down: Do not skip these. Before you begin your main activity, spend 5-10 minutes warming up with dynamic stretches that involve gentle, controlled movements through a full range of motion. Think arm circles, leg swings, torso twists, and walking lunges. This prepares your body for the work ahead. Afterward, spend another 5-10 minutes cooling down with static stretches, holding each stretch for 20-30 seconds to improve flexibility and aid recovery.

Listen with Compassion: Listening to your body means being willing to change or shorten a workout, or even take an unscheduled rest day, based on how you are genuinely feeling. This is not failure; it is intelligent self-regulation.

Doctor It Up #2: Maximize the FUN Factor-- Your Greatest Weapon for Consistency

This might sound obvious, but it is the secret that most fitness programs ignore. If an activity consistently feels like a burdensome chore, you have to drag yourself to, you will not stick with it long-term. Willpower is a finite resource. Joy is renewable.

Experiment Widely: Treat the menu of activities in the How-To section as a personal adventure. Try different things. Explore many settings. See what genuinely sparks your interest or makes you feel playful and free.

Doctor It Up #3: Make It Social--Amplify Connection & Accountability

As we will explore in depth in the next chapter, humans are deeply social creatures. We are wired for connection. Weaving social connection into your Green Exercise routine is a powerful strategy to amplify its benefits and make it more sustainable.

The Power of Shared Experience: A beautiful sunset is even more beautiful when shared with a friend. The challenge of a steep hill is reduced by having a workout buddy. Laughter and conversation can make the time fly by. Sharing your outdoor movement with people whose company you enjoy changes it from a solo task into a rewarding social event.

The Accountability Engine: Simple but powerful. It is much harder to skip a planned walk or run when you know a friend is waiting for you at the trailhead. This gentle, positive social pressure can be the deciding factor that gets you out the door on days when your motivation is low.

Your Mission: Proactively schedule active time with others. Suggest a walk-and-talk meeting with a colleague instead of a conference room. Create a weekly family tradition of an after-dinner stroll. Join a local hiking club or an outdoor fitness group.

Watercooler Fact:

Social Walking Bonus: Walking with a friend lowers blood pressure more than walking alone, thanks to oxytocin release.

Social walking lowers blood pressure more than solitary walking, because oxytocin is released when you're with people you like, and your fight-or-flight system is turned down. Group walks also improve sleep quality more than solitary ones. Walking with trusted others also improves sleep, and reduces sympathetic tone. Those benefits are partially mediated by oxytocin and the vagus. By making your movement social, you nourish your body and your social bonds simultaneously.

Doctor It Up #4: Stack Your Outdoor Rx Benefits

The Outdoor Rx steps are designed to work together. They are not isolated practices; they are interactive layers of medicine. Green Exercise provides the perfect platform for stacking multiple benefits into a single, efficient session.

Morning Sun (Chapter 1) + Movement: The ultimate morning routine. Take your daily dose of morning sunlight while you enjoy a brisk, invigorating walk or practice gentle outdoor yoga. This powerful combination sets your circadian rhythm, ignites your cortisol awakening response, and floods your system with endorphins, preparing you for a day of focused energy and positive mood.

Sky, Space, and Sea (Chapter 2) + Movement: This stack transforms your workout from a purely physical act into a potent mental and emotional reset. Intentionally choose a walking, running, or biking route that offers an expansive view of the sky or a distant horizon. As you move, your body gets the benefits of exercise, while your mind receives the awe-inspiring, perspective-shifting benefits we explored in Chapter 2. This is a powerful antidote to mental tunnel vision.

After your workout, use your cool-down period to perform the Horizon Scanning protocol. Find the farthest point you can see, let your gaze rest there, and allow your overworked eye muscles and your overstressed mind to relax completely. This practice quiets the ego, calms the nervous system, and solidifies the revitalizing effects of your movement.

Forest Bathing (Chapter 3) + Movement: While Forest Bathing is about slow, sensory immersion, you can incorporate its principles into your movement. During a slow walk or a rest break on a hike, intentionally practice the sensory invitations from Chapter 3. Listen deeply to the soundscape or notice the complex patterns of light and shadow. This moves a simple walk into a rich, mindful, and deeply restorative journey.

Winding Down with Darkness (Chapter 7) + Movement: A gentle, slow, and mindful evening stroll through your neighborhood as dusk falls can be a beautiful and highly beneficial part of your wind-down ritual. It helps your body transition away from the stress of the day and signals to your brain that it is time to prepare for a night of restful, restorative sleep.

Doctor It Up #5: Embrace Exercise Snacks

Banish the all-or-nothing thinking that so often derails our best intentions. You do not need a full hour to reap the benefits of movement. Shorter, more frequent bursts of purposeful movement throughout your day (what health experts call exercise snacks) absolutely count, and they add up to provide significant health benefits.

The 10-Minute Power Walk: A brisk 10-minute walk during your lunch break can improve your mood, clear your head, and help regulate your blood sugar after a meal.

The Stairwell Challenge: Make a conscious choice to take the stairs instead of the elevator. A few flights of stairs are a potent cardiovascular snack.

The Park Bench Circuit: While your kids are at the playground, use a nearby park bench to do a quick circuit of bodyweight exercises: 10 incline push-ups, 10 triceps dips, 20 step-ups. It only takes five minutes, and it matters.

Cultivating consistency with these smaller bouts of movement is often far more sustainable and ultimately more effective for busy people than relying only on infrequent, heroic workouts.

Your Outdoor Rx Action Space: Outdoor Motion Meter & Joyful Movement Journal

This Action Space is where you become the scientist of your own vitality. You'll track what you do, notice how it makes you feel, and find your own formula for joy and resilience in movement outside. You're gathering evidence to show Green Exercise belongs in your life. Open your Outdoor Rx notebook and begin.

My Outdoor Motion Meter & How I Felt Tracker

Date: _____

Time of Day I Moved My Body Outdoors: _____

Approx. Duration: _____ mins

My Chosen Outdoor Activity/Type of Movement Today: (Be specific--what did I choose to do with joy and intention?)

_____

Specific Location/Route: (Where did I experience the joy of outdoor movement today?)_____

Prevailing Weather/Environmental Conditions: (How did nature show up for me today?)_____

How My Movement Felt (My Personal "WIFM"-- Immediately AFTER the activity):_____

My Physical Body Feels: (e.g., Wonderfully Energized!, Pleasantly Fatigued but Stronger, More Relaxed and Open, Lighter and More Flexible)_____

My Mental/Emotional State Feels: (e.g., Noticeably Happier and More Optimistic!, Much Calmer and More Focused, Significantly Less Stressed, My Mind Feels Clearer)

_____

My Personal "Joy & Effort" Assessment (Rate 1-5, with 5 being the highest):

Enjoyment Factor Today: (1 = Felt like a total chore; 5 = Pure, unadulterated JOY!)

1 2 3 4 5

My Level of Perceived Exertion: (1 = Felt incredibly easy; 5 = Maximum effort for me today!)

1 2 3 4 5

My Reflections: Barriers Overcome/Solutions Found/Key Observations & Insights

Challenges & Solutions: What challenges did I face today (e.g., low motivation, bad weather, lack of time, physical discomfort)? How did I choose to handle those challenges with self-compassion and creativity?_____

_____

Key Observations: What specifically made this session especially enjoyable or meaningful (or less so)? Think about the specific details, sensory experiences or internal feelings that stood out._____

_____

Intention for Next Time: What is one small, actionable idea for making my next session even better, more consistent, or more enjoyable?_____

My Connection Meter:

Today's outdoor movement experience helped me to feel more deeply connected with: (Circle all that apply, or add your own words)

My Own Physical Body & Its Capabilities | The Beauty & Wonder of the Natural World | My Internal Source of Energy & Vitality | A Sense of Spontaneous Joy & Playfulness | Inner Calm & Mental Stillness | My Developing Strength & Resilience | A Cherished Friend, Loved One, or Pet | A

Heightened Sense of Presence & Mindfulness | Deep Feelings of Gratitude & Appreciation

The Big WIFM Question for Long-Term Success and Joyful Sustainability:

"As I continue this practice, am I noticing any consistent patterns in my personal levels of enjoyment, my daily energy, or my overall well-being that seem to be directly related to the specific type of outdoor activity I choose, the setting I'm in, the time of day I move, or whether I do it solo or in the company of others? Based on these emerging personal insights, how can I intentionally and creatively engineer more joyful, meaningful, and truly sustainable outdoor movement into the regular fabric of my weekly life?"

Chapter 5:
The Nature Connection: The Outdoors as Medicine for Isolation and Longevity

Introduction

Loneliness has doubled since 2000. Today, one in two Americans reports having three or fewer close friends. In the clinic, I see it written on the body: patients whose blood pressure is elevated, who have not slept well in a year, who feel exhausted for no clear reason, who are Vitamin D deficient, and who are slow to fight infections.

Loneliness raises dementia risk by up to 60% and shortens lifespan as powerfully as smoking 15 cigarettes a day. These are not abstract statistics. They are the lived symptoms of the Indoor Epidemic: social isolation as a biological stressor that drives chronic disease and accelerates aging.

> **Watercooler Fact:**
>
> **Outdoor Social Sleep Advantage**
>
> Walking with someone improves sleep quality more than exercising alone.

Fortunately, connection acts like medicine, and the outdoors makes it easier to take. Walking with a friend can lower systolic blood pressure by over 5 mmHg, a reduction equal to first-line drugs and stronger than walking alone. Outdoor conversations lower cortisol more than indoor ones. Even quietly sharing attention to something larger, a skyline, a flower garden, a stand of trees, reduces overactivity in the brain's Default Mode Network, easing repetitive rumination, stress, and depression.

These effects translate directly into longevity. People with stronger nature connections live healthier, with stronger bonds, less stress, and more sustainable habits, adding measurable life to those years. The prescription is simple: choose to go outside, move your body, and let nature do the rest.

Watercooler Fact:

Window Views Heal Faster

Hospital patients with a nature view use **22%** less opioid medication and leave **8%** earlier.

This chapter is your prescription to reconnect. Nature is not just a backdrop: it is an active partner. You'll see how outdoor settings make social connection easier, how they buffer the brain and body against chronic stress, and how simple practices such as farmers' markets, garden projects and horizon walks become powerful tools to repair both community and biology. Social cohesion regulates the nervous system, and nature amplifies its effect.

Digital Boundary Setup

- Use an analog alarm clock
- Keep your phone out of the bedroom
- Keep your journal by the bed
- Delay screens for the first 30 minutes of the day

The Healing Power of Human Connection Outdoors

Consider Dana, a 51-year-old patient who was the glue of her world: MVP at work, caregiver at home, leader of her church's community garden. Yet she herself was starving for connection. She spent more than 93% of her day inside, cycling between service, commuting, and collapsing in front of a screen. While people constantly surrounded her, her interactions were almost entirely transactional. She was giving, serving, solving, but receiving none of the reciprocal, restorative input her nervous system desperately needed.

The secret is simple: connect for real. Outdoor connection is a doctor's order because it taps into both biology and belonging. Whether with family, friends, pets, or neighbors, nature makes genuine presence easier. When you invite someone for a walk, a dog outing, or a trip to a farmers' market, you are not just socializing. You are lowering stress hormones, boosting immune function, and improving the metrics tied to longevity.

Nowhere is this more vivid than in children with Autism Spectrum Disorder (ASD). Loneliness in the modern age is not only an adult problem. It is often a shared family epidemic. When one person retreats into scrolling or gaming, the entire home absorbs the silence that follows. Parents and teens may sit in the same room, yet feel as if they are living separate lives shaped by separate screens. What looks like quiet is often unspoken disconnection, and over time it erodes the sense of belonging that every family needs.

The mission to reconnect begins with you. When you ask your teen to join you outside for a walk, a pickup game, or even reading on a blanket, you are doing more than offering time together. You are using shared attention to rebuild the social health of your family. Outdoor time becomes the medium through which presence returns and the Indoor Epidemic loses its grip.

Watercooler Fact:

Urban Antidepressant Trees

A **10%** increase in neighborhood tree canopy = **15% fewer antidepressant prescriptions**.

A 2023 JAMA Network Open report of 24 studies and over 700 children shows that outdoor, group-based therapies improved social communication, awareness, cognition, and motivation. Why?

Because nature softens the edges. A bird overhead, the crunch of leaves underfoot, or the rhythm of horseback riding creates shared points of attention that lower social pressure and build symbiosis. These programs didn't just reduce autistic mannerisms. They gave children the confidence to connect. Outdoors, nature becomes a co-therapist, helping to build resilience across a lifetime.

Your Mission: Connect Outdoors

If you feel the quiet ache of loneliness, even when your phone buzzes or you sit in a crowded room, know this: it is not weakness; it is biology. Your nervous system is signaling that it needs connection. And the most effective way to restore that connection is to go outside and share something real.

Here are practical, science-based ways to do it:

The Sky Picnic

Instead of another night indoors, carry dinner outside. Leave phones inside and sit together under the evening sky. Even a single hour reduces cortisol, lowers blood pressure, and helps reset circadian rhythms. A couple in their 40s who tried this simple sky picnic lowered their blood pressures and slept better within weeks. Shared awe turns routine meals into medicine.

The Horizon Hunt

Invite a friend: "I'm on a mission to find the best view in our neighborhood. Want to come scout?" Searching for a long sightline or the biggest patch of sky shifts perspective and reduces repetitive thought loops.

Watercooler Fact:

Horizon Focus Hack
Looking at distant vistas restores attention by **40%** after screen fatigue.

The horizon is more than scenery: it is therapy, training your brain to expand rather than contract.

The Sound Map

> **Watercooler Fact:**
>
> **Blue-Mindwaves Reset**
> Being near water shifts brainwaves into **Alpha/Theta**, the relaxed, creative states.

For the overstimulated or socially anxious, try this: sit back-to-back in a park and simply listen. Note each distinct sound (birdsong, leaves rustling, distant voices). Mapping sounds together pulls focus outward, lowers stress, and engages auditory pathways shown to improve cognitive function. Alignment grows quietly in the shared presence of sound.

The Nature Mandala

Gather leaves, stones, or twigs and create a temporary design together on the ground. No pressure, no permanence: just playful co-creation. Working side-by-side makes conversation easier and strengthens bonds through a low-stakes shared task. Creativity here is not about art, but about alignment.

The Farmers' Market Tour

Turn shopping into exploration. Walk through a local market and challenge each other to find the most unusual fruit or vegetable, then taste-test it together. Markets are third places or neutral spaces where community naturally forms. Novelty, laughter, and shared discovery strengthen bonds and, over time, reinforce social healthspan.

The Why: Why Getting Together Outdoors Is So Potent for Your Health, Your Happiness, and Even Your Longevity

Engaging in genuine and safe connections with others leads to the release of beneficial neurochemicals, most notably oxytocin, often called the bonding hormone.

Oxytocin is important for building feelings of trust, safety, empathy, generosity, and social bonding. When social cohesion occurs in natural environments, it reliably calms the body's physiological stress response, leading to lower levels of the stress hormone cortisol and reduced blood pressure and heart rate. This shift promotes a restorative rest-and-digest parasympathetic nervous system state, enhancing longevity.

This touches most of us. The feeling of loneliness--a quiet, persistent ache for deeper, more meaningful bonds--is not just in your head, and is not a sign of some personal failing. Loneliness is a significant, universal human experience and a fundamental biological signal from your ancient, evolved biology. And it's affecting more of us, more deeply, than perhaps ever before in human history.

Here are four ways nature and community can help heal loneliness:

1. The Modern Loneliness Problem

Surgeon General Murthy's advisory wasn't a document of vague concerns; it was a data-rich, science-backed wake-up call. It powerfully highlights that the absence of strong, consistent social connections carries significant, measurable, and often devastating health risks.

This statistic should stop each of us in our tracks: the Surgeon General's Advisory clearly states that the impact of measurable social disconnection on your risk for premature death can equal that of smoking up to 15 cigarettes a day. The science is blunt: a lack of real human resonance is a health hazard. This is a medical emergency for your heart, brain, and lifespan.

Let that sink in. The lack of something we often dismiss as a "nice-to-have," deep social bonding, is a mortality risk on par with a pack-a-day habit. The advisory meticulously documents that chronic loneliness is robustly associated with:

- A 29% increased risk of developing heart disease
- A 32% increased risk of having a stroke
- Significantly higher rates and earlier onset of debilitating anxiety disorders, major depressive episodes, and various forms of dementia, including Alzheimer's disease

Loneliness acts as a chronic, low-grade stressor, activating the body's fight-or-flight response system, relentlessly grinding your stress hormone system to overproduce constantly. As we've explored in Chapter 3, chronic cortisol elevation is measurably damaging, leading to a cascade of physical breakdowns. That includes dysregulated inflammation, the smoldering fire that underlies nearly every major modern disease. High cortisol levels elevate your blood pressure and strain your cardiovascular system. They also impair immune function, leaving you more vulnerable to illness.

> **Watercooler Fact:**
> **Loneliness = 15 Cigarettes:** Chronic loneliness carries the same mortality risk as smoking 15 cigarettes daily.

My patient Dana was in just this state. She had early osteoarthritis from hours in an office chair, weight gain from stress eating, and constant fatigue. Her burnout wasn't just a feeling of being tired; it was a state of physiological depletion driven by chronic, unbuffered stress.

With about one-in-two American adults reporting measurable levels of loneliness even before the pandemic further fractured our social ties, this isn't an individual issue. It is a critical and pervasive public health crisis that demands an urgent, compassionate, and creative response. And that's precisely where intentionally building meaningful connections, especially in the uniquely supportive embrace of nature, becomes such powerful and accessible medicine.

The modern ability to run your life without leaving the house comes with a hidden tax: isolation and minimal social skills. Nearly half of Gen Z say they often feel lonely, and depression and anxiety in young adults are rampant. Habits from screens bleed into face-to-face life. In personal interactions, there is silence where words should be, or a blank stare where symbiosis should spark. The idea that sitting on a bar stool to meet someone becomes novel. The more we live online, the less resilient our minds become and the more hollow our relationships feel. We are hyper-connected and deeply alone.

2. Nature's Social Magic: The Ultimate Social Lubricant

So, why does taking these important connections outdoors pack such an extra, uniquely beneficial punch? What is it about nature that makes it such a powerful ally in our quest for genuine human connection?

Have you ever noticed how conversations, even with people you don't know well, often seem to flow more easily, with less self-consciousness or awkwardness, when you're walking side-by-side in a park versus sitting directly face-to-face across a table? That's physiology as much as psychology.

Gentle movement and a shared view cue the vagus nerve that you're safe, which supports biological reciprocity. Eye contact, laughter, warm touch, and unhurried talk all stimulate oxytocin, which works with the vagus nerve's actions to lower stress and deepen trust.

Natural environments, by their very essence, provide a delightfully ever-changing supply of shared, neutral, and inherently interesting external focal points for your attention. It might be an unusual bird that flits across your path, a beautiful patch of wildflowers blooming along the trailside, or the sound of children laughing in the distance.

Readily available, non-personal subjects in nature make for wonderfully easy, organic conversation starters, like a display of gorgeous red peppers in the grocery store. They help bridge potential lulls in dialogue in a comfortable, natural way.

Critically, for many people who experience social anxiety, being outdoors significantly reduces the perceived pressure for constant, intense, direct eye contact, which can feel confrontational or scrutinizing in more formal indoor settings. The relaxed, spacious atmosphere promotes more open, spontaneous, and ultimately more authentic communication.

The Stress Melter x 2 Effect: A Potent Physiological Multiplier Effect

This is where true magic happens. When you combine the power of nature with positive social connection, you are giving your entire system a potent, double-whammy of stress reduction.

Dose #1: Nature's Calm. Your body responds to intentional time in most natural environments with a calmer physiology. That calm arrives through the vagus: rhythmic sounds, soft light, and gentle motion signal 'safe' and making interfacing with others easier. Nature exposure, as you now know, means lower levels of cortisol, lower blood pressure and heart rate, and a shift toward the restorative rest-and-digest mode of the parasympathetic nervous system.

Dose #2: Connection's Calm. When we bond genuinely with people we trust, the brain releases oxytocin, the bonding hormone, which reinforces the body's calming signal. Cortisol drops, heart rate steadies, and a sense of safety grows. The vagus nerve is at the center of this social engagement system, wiring us for eye contact, laughter, touch, and conversation.

When those cues show up outdoors, the effect grows. Natural sights and sounds help the vagus quiet the stress response and shift the body toward calm. Add real bonding, and oxytocin rises, reinforcing trust and bonding. Together, the two reinforce each other in a way that feels bigger than either alone. Outside, stress softens, conversations open up, and relationships deepen in ways that rarely happen in offices, cubicles, or restaurants.

Take Dana, for example. Her mind is always on call as she manages work, family, and everyone else's needs. But a simple protocol like the Sound Map with a friend could interrupt that loop. Instead of ruminating, her attention could shift outward to the birds, the breeze, even the layers of car sounds around her. Sitting side-by-side removes the pressure to perform (versus sitting face to face). Sitting with a trusted companion can help you load extra oxytocin to counterbalance the cortisol driving Dana's fatigue and stress eating. That's not just a pleasant outing. It's medicine.

3. Building Community Bonds & the Power of Third Places

This is where the magic of outdoor symbiosis ripples outward, from individual well-being to the health of an entire community. A significant body of research connects fields like environmental psychology, urban planning, and public health. The research consistently shows that communities blessed with accessible, safe, and well-used public parks, community gardens, and greenways usually exhibit demonstrably stronger, more resilient social ties among their residents.

Think about your own experience with third spaces. Where does community happen outside?

- It's the diverse group of dog owners striking up easy conversations while their pets play at the local dog park. Pets are fantastic social catalysts.

- It's the parents connecting and sharing support while watching their children play at the neighborhood playground.
- It's the neighbors of all ages and backgrounds enjoying a free outdoor concert or a community movie night in a central park.
- It's the vibrant, bustling energy of a local farmers' market, an important outdoor hub for community exchange between growers and eaters.
- It's the dedicated neighbors collaborating, learning, and building deep friendships while tending plots in a community garden.

This brings us back to the poignant irony of Dana's story. The community garden she founded is a perfect example of a thriving third place. It is a space designed for the thing she lacks: spontaneous, restorative, reciprocal social cohesion. The tragedy is that she views it as another part of her second place: another job to manage, another list of obligations. She helps others with this important hub, but is too depleted to benefit from it herself.

Dana's story is a powerful reminder that these third places only work their magic when we allow ourselves to be present and take part in them, not just administer them. These seemingly small, informal interactions are the threads that weave together the strong social fabric of a healthy, caring, and connected community.

4. The Equigenic Effect: Nature as a Strategy for Social Justice

Social justice is a critically important and often overlooked dimension of outdoor exchanges. An intriguing and rapidly growing body of research suggests that the health and well-being benefits of regular access to local green space are greatest and most impactful for populations and communities facing significant socioeconomic disadvantages and health inequities.

This powerful finding is sometimes called the equigenic effect of green space. The term means that equitable access to nature has the potential to help equalize health outcomes and actively reduce stark health disparities.

Here's why: Historically underserved, low-income, or disadvantaged neighborhoods often bear a greater burden of environmental stressors, such as noise and air pollution, and a lack of health-promoting resources, like safe parks and access to fresh food.

A safe, clean, and welcoming public park is not just a pleasant amenity; it is a powerful public health intervention. It provides a free and accessible place for stress reduction, physical activity, and social cohesion that may be absent elsewhere in the community. It directly buffers against the negative health impacts of the surrounding environment.

Ensuring truly equitable, safe, and community-driven access to high-quality parks, community gardens, and urban forests is not merely a nice-to-have civic goal. It is a direct pathway for promoting health equity. It is an important means of creating deeper social justice by addressing the historical inequities that have led to nature gaps between different communities. And ultimately, it is about collaboratively building healthier, more resilient, and more just communities for every single person.

The community garden Dana created is an equigenic force, whether she uses that term or not. By bringing a pocket of green, a source of healthy food, and a safe social space into her community, she has built a platform for health equity.

The final step in Dana's own healing journey would be to step down from her role as the tireless organizer and allow herself to become a simple participant. She could then receive the same medicine that she has so generously provided for everyone else.

The Compounding Interest of Alignment: Quality over Quantity

Alignment matters: A 23-year study of 553 adults found it isn't the size of your social circle that predicts your healthspan, but whether a few core relationships remain steady and supportive. Tracking self-rated health and depressive symptoms, researchers could detect no measurable benefit from having more friends.

What mattered was quality and stability: relationships that stayed reliable and deepened over the years. Biology rewards consistency, not quantity, freeing us from the pressure to be social butterflies.

The same study showed that occasional conflict or negative interactions don't derail long-term health. The body responds to the overall pattern, not every bump in the road. The task isn't to network endlessly or collect contacts, but to cultivate a few dependable bonds and allow them to strengthen. A quiet walk outdoors with one or two close friends is both fun and an investment in resilience and healthspan.

This conclusion was reinforced by a landmark 20-year study: the strongest predictor of long-term health was not cholesterol or blood pressure, but whether relationships remained stable and supportive.

Nature is the perfect setting for building those bonds. Outdoor spaces lower stress, quiet the brain's chatter, and make connecting easier. Your healthspan and longevity are not built on endless networking. They are built on consistent, caring bonding.

The How-To (Your Mission): Your Outdoor Connection Prescription

This section is your mission guide. Open the door to authentic engagements with others. Here are five ways to spark deeper relationships, outdoors:

1. Extend the Invitation: The Art of the Easy Yes

This is where it all begins: with a simple, thoughtful, human invitation. Don't just passively wait for resonance to appear magically. You must be the one to create the opportunity.

But how you invite someone is as important as the invitation itself. A vague, open-ended offer like "We should hang out sometime" isn't an invitation; it's a social burden. It puts all the planning pressure on the other person. A great invitation is the opposite: it's specific, it's appealing, and it makes saying "yes" feel easy and exciting.

The goal is to frame your invitation, so it lands not as another obligation on their already full plate, but as a welcome offer of a brief, refreshing respite. Keep it light, optional, and make it sound like something genuinely pleasant for both of you.

Scripts for Connection: Your Cut-and-Paste Guide

Here are specific scripts for different people in your life. Notice the formula: Acknowledge them + Specific, low-stakes outdoor plan + An easy, judgment-free out.

For a Colleague You'd Like to Know Better:

Don't Say: "Want to get lunch sometime?" (Vague, puts them on the spot).

Try This: "I've been feeling so drained from all these Zoom meetings. I'm planning to eat my lunch outside in that little courtyard for 20 minutes tomorrow to get some sun. I'd love the company if you're free and want to join."

Why It Works: It's a defined, short timeframe. It has a clear benefit for you (getting sun), which removes the pressure from them to be endlessly entertaining. It's a join me if you can offer, not a demand. This is a perfect way to repurpose a solitary desk lunch into an alignment snack.

For a Friend You Haven't Seen in Ages:

Don't Say: "We are so overdue! We have to catch up soon!" (Expresses desire but creates no action).

Try This: "Hey [Name], I was just thinking about you and our old hiking trips. I'm planning a very easy, 30-minute walk around [local park/lake] on Saturday morning just to clear my head. Would you be up for joining me for some fresh air and a chat? No worries at all if the timing is bad, but I'd love to see you."

Why It Works: It references a shared positive memory, which strengthens the existing bond. It defines the time and effort (easy, 30-minute walk), making it feel manageable. The no-worries clause gives them a graceful way to decline without feeling guilty, which paradoxically makes them more likely to say yes or suggest an alternative.

For a Neighbor You Only Wave To:

Don't Say: "Hi." (And keep walking).

Try This (The Micro-Invitation): "Morning! I'm about to have my coffee on the front steps for 10 minutes to soak up this amazing sun. Feel free to say hi on your way out if you have a second."

Why It Works: This is the lowest-stakes invitation possible. It requires nothing from them but a brief chat. You are anchoring the activity to something you're already doing, making it feel spontaneous and casual. These brief weak-tie interactions are incredibly powerful for building a background sense of community and safety.

For a Family Member (to Break a Routine):

Don't Say: "What do you want to do this weekend?" (Opens the door to decision fatigue and defaulting to screens).

Try This: "Instead of our usual Sunday afternoon TV marathon, I have a different idea. I found a trail along the [local creek/waterfront] that I've never explored. Let's grab a coffee to go and just walk for 45 minutes and see what's there. My treat."

Why It Works: It offers a new alternative to a stale routine. It removes the burden of planning from them. It frames the activity as a small adventure or discovery, making it more appealing.

This is a skill Dana must learn. She is a master of the grand gesture: organizing the entire garden, running the fundraiser. But she has forgotten how to make the small, reciprocal invitation. Her healing begins not by hosting a potluck for 20, but by asking one person, "I'm going to the garden just to watch the sunset for 15 minutes. Want to join me?" It is a shift from serving to sharing.

> **Watercooler Fact:**
>
> Regular nature exposure **reduces cardiovascular disease risk by up to 12%** and **lowers resting heart rate by an average of 3-4 beats per minute**.

2. Choose the Venue: Curating Your Connecting Space

When you're planning to connect with others outdoors, thoughtfully selecting a location is critical. The right venue can make or break the experience. The goal is to choose an environment where everyone can feel genuinely relaxed, safe, and fully at ease, so they can connect authentically.

Think like a film director setting a scene. What is the mood you want to create? Relaxed and contemplative? Playful and energetic? Your options are often far more plentiful than you might first imagine, even in a dense urban environment. But beyond aesthetics, you must consider the practicalities.

Your Venue Selection Checklist:

- Convenience: How close is the location to everyone's home or workplace? Is parking easy, or is it reachable via public transport? Removing logistical hurdles is key.
- Amenities: Are there clean and accessible restrooms? Are there comfortable benches or other seating options? Is there drinking water available? Is there shade from the sun or shelter from a light rain? Thinking ahead about these details shows care.
- Ambiance & Safety: What's the general atmosphere? Is it a loud, busy park or a quiet, tranquil garden? What is the perceived safety of the place, especially at the time of day you're planning to meet?
- Accessibility: This is not up for debate. Can everyone you're inviting comfortably and safely navigate the space?

Tailoring the Venue to Your Guests:

For Someone with Mobility Challenges: Don't guess. Ask. "I was thinking we could go to [park name]. Do you know if their paths are pretty flat and paved?" Choose locations that offer relatively smooth, even paths and readily available, sturdy benches, preferably with backrests. Many botanical gardens, university campuses, and newer city parks are designed with accessibility in mind.

For a Friend with Young Children: The goal is alignment for the adults, but the kids need to be safe and engaged. A park with a playground next to a comfortable seating area is perfect. Or choose a natural area with engaging features: a small creek to splash in, interesting rocks to climb, a wide-open field to run in. This allows the kids to play while you connect.

For Someone with Sensory Sensitivities: A bustling park on a Saturday might be overwhelming. Suggest a quieter venue or time. This could be a weekday morning walk, a visit to a less-frequented pocket park, a lower key community garden during open hours, or even a local cemetery, which are sometimes beautifully landscaped and peaceful (again, if such spaces feel safe).

Under-the-Radar Connection Spots:

- University Campuses: Often beautifully maintained, open to the public, and full of benches, gardens, and interesting architecture.
- Hospital Gardens: Many hospitals have created healing gardens that are incredibly peaceful and designed for restoration. They are often quiet, accessible, and underutilized by the public.
- Public Plazas with Water Features: The sound of a fountain can create a natural privacy bubble, allowing for intimate conversation even in a bustling public square.
- Well-Lit Riverwalks or Beach Paths in the Evening: A post-dinner walk can feel magical and is a great way to wind down the day together.

3. Set the Stage for Presence: The Gentle Digital Detox

You've extended the perfect invitation and chosen a great location. Now for the most critical step: creating a space for genuine, undivided attention. In the modern world, this means consciously addressing the tyranny of the screen.

Our phones are attention thieves. The constant pings, notifications, and the reflexive urge to just check one thing can fragment our focus and dilute the quality of our most important interactions. Gently and collaboratively suggesting a brief digital detox is not about being preachy or rigid; it's about co-creating a protected space for real connection. It's a gift you give each other.

How to Gently Suggest Unplugging:

The key is to be collaborative and frame it as a mutual benefit.

The Brain Break Approach: "To give our brains a break from all the usual screen demands, what do you think about us both putting our phones away and putting them on silent just for this little while?"

The Protect Our Time Approach: "I'm so looking forward to just catching up. How about we make this a phone-free zone for our picnic, so that we can connect without interruptions?"

The Lead by Example Approach: As you meet up, simply put your own phone on silent and place it in your pocket or bag, saying, "Okay, I'm putting my phone away so I can give you my full attention. You have it!" Often, the other person will follow suit without you even having to ask.

Navigating Resistance with Grace:

What if your friend is a doctor on call, or a parent waiting for a call from a babysitter? Don't be a zealot. The goal is connection, not conflict.

Suggest a Compromise: "Of course! How about we just put them on vibrate and agree only to check them if it's the specific call you're waiting for? That way we can still tune out the other noise."

Remember, the goal isn't a perfect, distraction-free bubble. It's the shared intention to be present that matters. In a world that steals our attention 93% of the time, that shared intention to be present is a remarkable act. Often, simply showing up for each other, with genuine warmth and openness, and sharing quiet time in a supportive, natural environment is the most restorative part of the entire experience. For Dana, whose phone is a relentless tether to others' needs, putting it away for 30 minutes is a deliberate act of self-care and boundary-setting. It is the first step in signaling to herself and her friend that this time is different. This time is for her.

4. The Art of Outdoor Conversation: Listening, Sharing, and Savoring Silence

Once you are together in your chosen outdoor space, with distractions minimized, you can engage in a higher quality conversation. Connection is a two-way street, built on a foundation of both generous listening and authentic sharing.

Practice Active, Compassionate Listening:

This is perhaps the greatest and most healing gift you can offer another human. It is more than not talking. It is an active, engaged process.

Ask Open-Ended Questions: Go beyond the superficial. Instead of "How was your week?" (which invites a one-word answer), try a question that invites reflection and feeling: "How has this week been feeling for you?" or "What's been taking up most of your headspace lately?"

Listen with Your Whole Being: Put away your own internal to-do list and truly tune in. Don't just wait your turn to speak. Listen to understand, not just reply. Use affirming nonverbal cues: nod, maintain comfortable eye contact, and orient your body toward them.

Reflect What You Hear: A powerful technique is to paraphrase their feelings back to them. "Wow, it sounds like you're feeling incredibly frustrated by that situation at work," or "It sounds like you felt really proud of that moment." This shows you are hearing their words and understanding their emotional core.

Share Authentically and Reciprocally:

Meaningful connection requires mutual self-disclosure. Be willing to share your own thoughts, feelings, and experiences appropriately. This builds shared humanity and deepens trust. However, be mindful not to dominate the conversation or turn it into a monologue. Aim for a comfortable, balanced give-and-take, where both people feel seen and heard.

Embrace the Outdoor Silence:

One of the most significant differences between indoor and outdoor conversation is the nature of silence. Indoors, a lull in conversation can feel awkward, like a void that needs to be filled. Outdoors, silence feels different. It feels shared. The rustle of leaves, a distant birdsong, the rhythm of your own footsteps are gentle environmental sounds, and fill the space.

Don't fear these quiet moments. They are often where the deepest connection happens. It's in the shared, unspoken appreciation of a view, the comfortable companionship of walking side-by-side without needing to speak. It's a quiet acknowledgment that your presence together is enough.

5. Use the Environment as Your Co-facilitator

Don't let the beauty and aliveness of your natural surroundings be merely a passive backdrop. Make a conscious, joyful effort to engage with the environment together. Let nature become an active, engaging, and wonderfully inspiring co-participant in your interaction.

How to Make Nature an Active Participant:

Point Out Specifics: Actively share what you notice. "Wow, look at the iridescent shimmer on that dragonfly's wings!" "Did you hear that hawk just now?" These shared observations subtly build rapport and create a 'we're in this together' feeling.

Share Sensory Experiences: Engage all the senses. "This breeze carrying the scent of pine feels absolutely amazing, doesn't it?" or "The fragrance of the forest floor after that light rain is just incredible." This grounds both of you in the present moment.

Let It Spark Curiosity: Use the environment as a source of endless, non-threatening conversation starters. "I wonder what kind of tree that is." "Look how the ants are working together to carry that leaf." This external focus is a huge relief from the pressure of purely internal or personal topics, especially in new or developing relationships.

Shared, multi-sensory, embodied experiences like watching the ants can be incredibly bonding. You're not just interacting with each other in a social vacuum; you're actively and joyfully interacting with and within a living environment together.

For Dana, the community garden had become a place of duty, a list of tasks. By inviting a friend to join her there not to work, but simply to find the most beautiful flower, to watch the bees, to taste a ripe tomato right off the vine together, she could change her relationship with the space. It would cease to be a second place of work and become a third place of restoration and connection. The environment itself, which she had viewed as a project to be managed, could finally become her partner in healing.

Helpful Tips and Bonus Info

These ideas are for anyone who wants to deepen real-world connection but isn't sure where to start or who feels awkward about small talk. Social bonds, particularly when forged outdoors, improve healthspan by activating brain pathways of safety, belonging, and well-being, which are antidotes to the biological toll of loneliness.

Nature Note: The Unifying Power of Shared Purpose

If direct conversation feels daunting, try centering connection on a shared outdoor activity. Purpose is a powerful bonding agent. It shifts the focus from "What are we going to talk about?" to "What are we going to do together?" This side-by-side engagement allows conversation to emerge naturally, without pressure.

Volunteer Together: Shared purpose is a potent connector. Don't just go for a walk in a park; join a park cleanup day. Don't just admire a community garden; sign up for a two-hour volunteer slot together. Working alongside someone for a cause you both believe in, like clearing an invasive species, planting native flowers or harvesting apples for a local food bank, builds a unique and powerful camaraderie. You connect through shared effort and accomplishment.

Learn Something New Together: Shared discovery is invigorating. Instead of just walking a familiar path, sign up for a guided nature walk with a local naturalist. Take an outdoor class on bird identification, nature photography, or even responsible wild foraging (always with an expert to ensure safety). The shared experience of being novices, of learning and asking questions, breaks down social barriers and gives you an endless supply of things to talk about.

Create Something Together: When you work on something creative together outdoors like building a birdhouse, creating land art, or sketching together, you activate your parasympathetic nervous system. You also allow your nervous system to cool down, and that actually deepens social connection. Focusing on the activity rather than forcing conversation, your brain takes away the stress response it normally prepares for socializing. If you're lucky, an authentic bonding occurs.

> **Watercooler Fact:**
> **Green Space Prescription:** 120 minutes per week in nature is the minimum effective dose for significant health benefits.

Play Together: As adults, we forget how to play. Reclaim it. Play is a language of pure connection. A casual game of frisbee or catch, a friendly round of bocce ball, or even just skipping stones on a pond, stream or lake can dissolve stress and inhibition. Laughter is a direct pathway to bonding, and outdoor play gives you the space to find it.

Doctor It Up! Overcoming Connection Hurdles

Even with the best intentions, real-world barriers can get in the way. Here are my clinical strategies for overcoming the most common hurdles to outdoor connection.

For the Shy or Socially Anxious: If social interaction triggers your sympathetic nervous system (again, your fight-or-flight response) the evidence-based approach is to externalize focus, which takes your nervous system out of high alert. Start small, start simple, and start with someone you already trust. Choose activities where the environment itself is the star of the show.

Strategy: The Parallel Play Protocol. Think of how young children play. They often engage in parallel play, doing the same activity together without intense interaction. You can adapt this. Invite a friend for birdwatching. The focus is on the birds, not generating witty banter. Go to an outdoor concert or movie. You are sharing an experience, side-by-side, without the need for constant conversation. The shared external focus provides a comfortable buffer, allowing connection to happen organically.

For the Overly Busy (The Connection Snack Protocol): In our chronically over-scheduled lives, finding a two-hour block for socializing can feel impossible. If that's your reality, don't give up. Shift your focus to high-quality connection snacks: shorter, intentional interactions that still deliver a powerful dose of well-being.

Strategy 1: The Walk-and-Talk Phone Call. Change an ordinary phone call with a friend or family member into a more engaging, powerful experience. Agree to both step outside and walk during the call, even if you're in different cities. The gentle movement and fresh air will energize both of you, making the conversation feel more dynamic and less like just another task on your to-do list.

Strategy 2: The Commute Detour. If you and a colleague work near each other, suggest a 15-minute detour on your commute. Instead of heading straight to your cars or the subway, take a short, designated walk together through a nearby park or plaza to decompress from the workday before heading your separate ways. It's a transitional ritual that provides a powerful buffer between your work life and home life.

For Differing Abilities or Interests: If you want to connect with someone whose physical energy levels, mobility, or interests differ from your own, the key is flexibility and a focus on presence over performance.

Strategy: The Hub-and-Spoke Plan. Choose a location that acts as a comfortable hub and offers various spokes of activity. For example, meet at an accessible public park with a comfortable bench overlooking a pleasant view (the hub). One person might prefer to sit and chat, while the other takes a more vigorous walk along a nearby path (the spoke), returning to the hub to reconnect. You can still share the beginning and end of the experience. The focus should always be on the quality of your presence with each other, not on perfectly matched activity levels. Remember, the most meaningful connections often happen in the simplest, most unforced moments of just being peacefully together in a supportive, natural space.

The Resolution: Dana Remembers Herself

For weeks after our conversation, nothing changed for Dana. The weight of her obligations felt too immense, adding one more thing, even something for herself, felt impossible. The cycle of service and exhaustion continued. Her back pain and stress eating persisted.

The turning point didn't come from a grand resolution. It came from a moment of quiet desperation. One Tuesday evening, after a grueling day, she was standing in her kitchen, scrolling through her phone, fielding texts about garden watering schedules and a potluck she was supposed to be organizing. She felt the familiar throb begin behind her right eye. She looked out the window at the community garden (the one she had poured her life into) and felt a deep sense of resentment. It was another job, another mouth to feed.

At that moment, she remembered our conversation about connection snacks and the art of the easy yes. She thought of the Tasting Tour protocol. On an impulse, she texted a single person, a quiet woman from her church named Maria, who she knew was recently widowed.

Her text was specific, low-pressure, and didn't ask for any work. "Hi Maria. This is Dana. I'm heading over to the garden in 10 minutes, not to work, but just to taste what's ripe. I'm on a mission to find the single best-tasting cherry tomato. Could you be my fellow judge? No obligation at all."

Maria replied almost instantly: "I'd love that."

That evening, for the first time in over a year, Dana walked into the garden with no agenda other than her own simple, sensory pleasure. She and Maria walked the rows, not pulling weeds, but searching for the darkest red tomatoes. They picked them straight from the vine, the sun still warm on their skin, and tasted them right there, laughing as the juice ran down their chins. They debated the merits of Sun Golds versus Sweet

Millions. They talked, not about church business or their problems, but about the taste of summer.

The conversation was easy, flowing along as they walked. The setting sun, the scent of basil, the shared, simple purpose all made it a perfect Stress Melter. Dana felt the tension in her lower back begin to unclench. For twenty minutes, she wasn't the MVP or the glue. She was just Dana, a woman tasting tomatoes with a friend. When she got home, she realized with a start that the throb in her head was gone.

This small, successful experiment emboldened her. The next week, she delegated the potluck planning to someone else. Instead, she invited another friend to join her for a Sound Map session on a bench in the garden, just listening to the evening sounds.

Slowly, she began to change her relationship with the space. It gradually ceased to be her second job and became her sanctuary. She started hosting informal harvest and chat sessions, where the only goal was for a few people to pick whatever was ready and enjoy each other's company.

Dana didn't quit her roles. She didn't stop being the helpful, caring person she was. But she learned to create connections differently. She learned to make small, reciprocal invitations that nourished her as much as they did others. She learned that true connection wasn't about serving everyone, but about sharing a genuine, present moment with someone. By stepping back from being the manager and allowing herself to become a participant, Dana finally began to receive the healing medicine of the community she had built.

Your Outdoor Rx Action Space: Outdoor Connection Log & Relationship Nourisher

Use your Outdoor Rx notebook to document your journey. By consciously tracking your efforts and reflecting on your experiences, you train your brain to notice and focus on what truly matters for your health and happiness. You are not just fighting your own loneliness; you are weaving a stronger social fabric for yourself and those you care about.

My Shared Time Outdoors Rx Log: Tracking My Journey to Deeper Connection

Date: _____

Approximate Time of Day & Duration: _____ mins/hours

With Whom Did I Intentionally Connect Today? (Be specific. Note their name and your relationship, e.g., "My friend, Sarah," "My son, Leo," "My neighbor from across the hall, John," "A new acquaintance from my yoga class.")

_____

Specific Location & Our Shared Outdoor Activity: (Paint a picture. What was the protocol or activity? Where did nature host you? e.g., "A Horizon Hunt at Hilltop Park," "A tasting tour at the Saturday Farmer's Market," "A simple walk-and-talk along the river path.")

_____

A Highlight Moment or Particularly Positive Feeling from This Interaction: (What specific moment, shared glance, burst of laughter, or quiet sense of understanding made your heart feel a little warmer or lighter? e.g., "The moment we both spotted the hawk circling overhead," "Laughing about how sour the wild berries were," "The comfortable silence while we watched the sunset.")_____

_____

How Did the OUTDOOR Setting Specifically Enhance Our Connection? (Take a moment to really consider this. Did it feel more relaxed than meeting indoors? Was it easier to talk while walking side-by-side? Did the natural sounds fill the silences comfortably? Did a shared observation of nature provide an easy conversation starter or a moment of shared wonder?)_____

My General Feeling/Mood & Energy Level Before This Connection: (Briefly note your state before the interaction, e.g., "Stressed and rushed from work," "Felt tired and a bit disconnected," "Mind was scattered.")

_____

My General Feeling/Mood & Energy Level After This Connection (The Benefit!): (Note any positive shifts, e.g., "Feeling so much lighter and happier," "My stress has melted away," "Felt more seen and understood," "My energy actually picked up.")

_____

Nourishing My Connections & Planning for More

One specific thing I appreciated about the person I was with today: (e.g., "Their great sense of humor," "The thoughtful way they listened," "Their willingness to try something new.")

_____

How did this outdoor connection feel qualitatively different or more enriching than a typical indoor interaction? (What was the unique magic ingredient that being outdoors seemed to add for you and for your connection? e.g., "Less pressure," "More spontaneous," "Felt more like a shared adventure.")

_____

(Your Next Mission) What is one small, concrete, and actionable idea for a future shared outdoor activity? (Be specific: What is the activity/protocol? With whom might I share it? When, realistically, could I take the first step, even if it's just sending the invitation?)_____

_____

Your Personal Benefit Statement for a More Connected Life:

Reflect on this powerful prompt to solidify your intention: Thinking about the vital importance of connection for my health and happiness, as emphasized by the U.S. Surgeon General, who in my life (including myself!) might benefit most from a thoughtful invitation to spend some simple, quality time outdoors together this week? What is one small, low-pressure, creative outdoor invitation I can courageously and warmly extend today or tomorrow?_____

_____

Chapter 6:
Gardening Rx: Cultivating Your Longevity from Soil to Plate

Introduction: The Mission to Grow Your Health from the Ground Up

Ever felt that primal satisfaction of plunging your hands into cool, loamy soil? The joy of watching a seed you planted unfold into life? The satisfaction of eating something you grew?

Gardening offers more than beauty or food. Mindful, repetitive actions like planting, watering, weeding and harvesting lower cortisol, activate the parasympathetic nervous system, and may even help protect telomeres. It is no coincidence that across the Blue Zones, where people live the longest and have the greatest healthspan, gardening is a universal practice.

> **Watercooler Fact:**
>
> **Soil Biodiversity:** One teaspoon of healthy garden soil has more microorganisms than there are people on Earth.

The secret starts in the soil. Healthy soil isn't dirt: soil is *alive*. Every handful is a pharmacy of microbes, including species like Mycobacterium vaccae, which can boost serotonin and temper inflammation as you work the soil. Regenerative practices such as reduced tillage, diverse cover crops, and rich compost feed those microbes; the microbes feed the plants, and the plants feed you and your own microbiome. Your garden becomes part of that healing loop.

When you garden organically, avoiding synthetic artificial chemical pesticides, herbicides and fungicides, you multiply those benefits. You're not just protecting your own health and that of anyone else who might eat what you grow; you're also safeguarding pollinators, birds, other animals, and the water supply. You're reducing indoor contamination from pesticide drift in the air and on your shoes and clothes.

Organic gardening keeps toxic residues out of your food, your home, the air, soil, and water supply. It is one of the most vital choices you can make for both your health and everyone else's.

Kitchen Detox Checklist

- Remove scented candles
- Use a HEPA-filter in bedrooms
- Avoid storing pesticides indoors
- Choose fragrance-free laundry detergents

That choice is even more consequential in a world of modern 'vectors' such as pesticide residues in food, solvents in water, pollutants in air and elsewhere.

Research shows that the herbicide paraquat may contribute to Parkinson's disease alongside other risks; laboratory models even use paraquat to induce neurodegeneration. Similarly, glyphosate (N- (phosphonomethyl) glycine), the active ingredient in Roundup, has been linked in some studies to endocrine disruption, microbiome changes, and possible carcinogenic effects. While the E.P.A. still allows both paraquat and glyphosate in the U.S., paraquat is banned in the EU, China, and Brazil, and glyphosate is restricted in some nations in the EU and the Gulf Region.

Similar patterns have played out with lead paint, endocrine disruptors (including some flame retardants, phthalates, PFAS), and some additives to food and cosmetics. Choosing organic and low-toxin practices isn't perfectionism and can't be perfect. But reducing your risk to your brain, your other organs, and especially to young bodies across your lifespan is prudent and non-negotiable preventive health.

The Indoor Epidemic thrives on disconnection from food, from soil, from natural cycles. Gardening is its antidote.

> **Watercooler Fact:**
>
> **Myopia Prevention Dose**
>
> Children who spend **2+ hours/day** outdoors halve their risk of nearsightedness (**50% reduction**).

Gardens restore what has been lost. In a school garden, children learn from the natural world itself. They experiment, problem-solve, and work with living systems rather than screens. I wish every school made growing food a regular class, from tending vegetables and berries to composting and saving seeds.

> **Watercooler Fact:**
>
> **Outdoor Recess = Vision Protection**
> Boosting recess time cut new myopia cases from **17.65%** → **8.41%** in a year.

This kind of hands-on education anchors children in something real and gives them the grounding that an online life cannot provide.

The Indoor Epidemic

Americans now spend over **90%** of their time indoors, with the average adult getting less than 1 hour of outdoor time per day.

93%	**7h**	**50%**
Indoor Time	Screen Time	Increase
Percentage of time the average American spends indoors	Daily recreational screen time for average adult	Rise in indoor time since 1990s

This dramatic shift in our environment is changing our relationship with exercise in unexpected ways.

Indoor classrooms can become filtered environments that separate students from the sensory richness of the real world. The practical skills that build patience and resilience begin to fade. But gardening as part of the curriculum, as Alice Waters has championed for decades, teaches more than just the senses.

Every time you lean over a potted herb, touch its soil, or taste something you grew, you're interrupting the cycle of sitting, scrolling, and sanitizing that erodes your health indoors.

Consider my patient, Greg. At 36, he's a world-builder of model everything. His apartment is filled with miniature trains, perfectly scaled landscapes, and entire model cities constructed with painstaking precision. His safe place. A world he controls down to the last millimeter, because the world outside his window is messy.

"I don't do bugs," Greg explained during our first virtual visit. "Or heat. Or noise. Or strangers. Or humidity. Or basically anything involving outdoors."

Raised on indoor hobbies and sustained by a work-from-home coding job, Greg rarely steps outside. He orders everything online. His longest walk is to the mailbox ten feet outside his door. He'd been warned about rising blood pressure and low Vitamin D levels. Intentionally going outside for this, never mind gardening, feels absurd. Threatening, even.

For Greg and for others insulated from the earth Gardening Rx is the perfect bridge. A way to engage with nature on our terms. Small, controlled, deeply rewarding.

Your Mission, Should You Choose to Dig In

Your mission is clear: cultivate life. It could be a few herbs on a windowsill, a pot of greens on a balcony, a corner of backyard soil, or a shared plot in a community garden. The form doesn't matter. What matters is choosing to nurture something green and alive.

> **Watercooler Fact:**
>
> **Longevity in 4 Minutes**
> Just **4.4 minutes/day** of vigorous outdoor movement cuts premature death by **26–30%**.

Gardening is a systematic practice of well-being: preparing soil, planting seeds, watering, weeding, and harvesting. Each step lowers stress, restores perspective, and feeds resilience. The payoff is far greater than the effort: more energy, calm, and clarity than you started with.

Here's the truth no one tells you: the tomatoes are a bonus. The real harvest is perspective. Instead of chasing deadlines, you're watching leaves unfurl. Instead of doom-scrolling, you're outsmarting aphids. Hands in the soil clear the mind in ways modern life can't.

Gardening is medicine for longevity: it delivers flavor and nutrition, and also purpose, grounding, and connection to life's oldest rhythms. That sense of meaning and continuity fuels resilience across decades and makes the garden among the most effective longevity tools you have.

The Why: Why Getting Dirty Is Powerful Medicine

The simple, ancient act of gardening is a conversation with the earth. Modern science now confirms this as remarkably potent, multifaceted medicine. The range of scientifically documented benefits is astonishing, touching nearly every part of human well-being.

What feels like a simple hobby is actually a cascade of powerful, positive physiological and psychological events, starting with the soil, its relationship to the microbiome, effect on inflammation, your mind, your body and then your food.

1. Soil Isn't Just 'Dirt': A Living, Breathing Ecosystem

We need to reframe what we call the ground beneath our feet. What you might call dirt is often really soil: Earth's original, well-stocked kitchen and kitchen medicine cabinet. As a trained chef who has had the privilege of cooking in a Michelin-starred farm-proud restaurant, calling soil dirt would never fly.

Soil has all the magic of a vibrant ecosystem packed with invisible allies for your gut, mood, and immune system. And as a regenerative farmer who loves getting his hands dirty, I can tell you that dirt is dead, and that healthy soil is a living, active, biological super-organism that's the foundation of all terrestrial life.

A single teaspoon of healthy garden soil contains billions of bacteria and more individual organisms than there are humans on Earth. It holds miles of thread-like fungal hyphae, a dazzling array of archaea, protozoa, and countless other microbes, all interacting in an intricate dance of symbiosis and nutrient cycling.

This Is the Soil's Microbiome

These organisms are the world's true farmers. They convert raw minerals and decaying organic matter into bioavailable nutrients plants need to thrive. Specialized bacteria fix atmospheric nitrogen, making it usable. Vast underground networks of mycorrhizal fungi act as a sophisticated wood-wide web, connecting different plants' root systems to share nutrients, water, and even defense signals about pests and diseases.

This living matrix is what Greg so desperately avoided. His entire life was built as a fortress against the messy and unpredictable. His meticulously crafted miniature worlds were sterile, controllable, and clean. His fear of dirt was, at its core, a fear of this teeming, uncontrolled microscopic life.

Yet the thing he perceived as contamination is actually a foundational source of health.

The rich, earthy aroma of healthy soil comes from bacteria called Actinomycetes and is literally the scent of life at work. Healthy, biologically active soil is not a given, by any means: it must be nurtured and built. On my farm, we try to achieve it through practices such as no-till, cover cropping, and adding organic, biologically active supplements and fertilizers. When soil is nurtured in this way, it not only improves the quality of the food and also supports our own microbiota, from the gut to the skin.

Recognizing soil not as a threat but as a vital, living partner is the first step toward understanding Gardening Rx's power.

Our hyper-sanitized lives have stripped away microbial diversity, leaving many of us with what scientists call a microbial desert. Yet your gut microbiome, your vast internal ecosystem of healthful microbes, evolved to thrive on constant input from soil, plants, and the natural world.

> **Watercooler Fact:**
> A healthy gut contains over 100 trillion microbes, including bacteria, viruses, and fungi. While the exact number varies, this diverse community is vital for functions like digestion, vitamin absorption, and immune defense.

Gardening is one of the most direct ways to restore that connection. As you work the soil, beneficial microbes transfer to your skin and under your nails, enriching your external microbiome and strengthening barrier defenses. Some of these organisms are carried incidentally into your body through touch and the food you grow, where they help reseed your gut ecosystem. Eating homegrown, minimally processed foods delivers even greater microbial diversity right where it matters most.

This diversity matters because your gut is not just for digestion: it's your second brain. The gut-brain axis, carried by the vagus nerve, transmits microbial signals to your central nervous system. Your gut produces short-chain fatty acids like butyrate and neurotransmitter precursors like tryptophan. These compounds regulate mood, stress, and inflammation.

Your gut produces more serotonin than your brain, much of it made by microbes. Richer microbial diversity means more balanced neurotransmitter production. The result: steadier mood and a calmer, more resilient brain.

The result: Richer microbial diversity means more balanced neurotransmitter production, steadier vagal tone and calmer, more resilient brain chemistry. This is one of medicine's most exciting frontiers. Your mental health is literally rooted in the health of the soil you touch.

3. Training Your Immune System (The 'Old Friends' Hypothesis)

This vital microbial exchange is central to a crucial concept in modern immunology: the Old Friends Hypothesis (see Glossary).

Here's the theory: human immune systems co-evolved over millennia in environments teeming with diverse microorganisms from soil, water, and plants. Regular, lifelong exposure to these largely harmless Old Friends is fundamental for proper development, education, and calibration of our immune systems.

This microbial exposure fundamentally trains the immune system, teaching crucial lessons in tolerance. It helps the immune system learn to distinguish genuine threats (such as pathogenic viruses) from harmless substances (such as pollen or food proteins).

However, our modern, overly sanitized, indoor-centric lifestyles may inadvertently lead to an immune system that is untrained, dysregulated, or simply bored. Without its old microbial friends to interact with, the immune system can become more prone to overreacting. It can launch attacks against harmless allergens, leading to allergies and asthma, or mistakenly attack the body's own healthy tissues, resulting in autoimmune diseases.

In addition, something big just shifted in how we understand the immune system, which we've long known can influence brain function. Think fever fog, inflammation-linked depression, even long COVID. The gut-brain-immune connection is emerging as central to longevity, and we're just beginning to decode the messages.

Recent longevity research tracking over 45,000 people for 17 years found something striking: the slowest-aging organs weren't the heart or liver but the brain and the immune system. People whose brains and immune systems aged more slowly lived longer, and when both aged slowly together, the benefit was even greater.

What does this have to do with gardening? Everything. Gardening immerses you in a diverse microbial ecosystem, especially in healthy soil, which trains your immune system through your skin, lungs, and gut. This low-dose microbial training tempers inflammation, curbs immune overreaction, and sharpens your body's ability to identify real threats, like infection or cancer. Because your immune system is deeply intertwined with your brain, this microbial training may also slow brain aging and help preserve thinking ability. In short, gardening feeds your body with immune-brain resilience, which extends your healthspan.

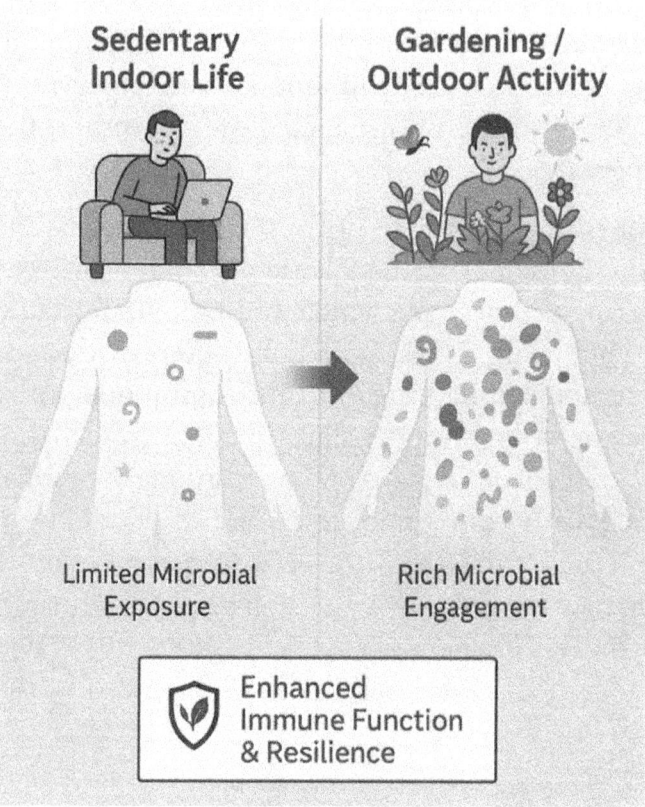

Gardening, with its inherent, joyful contact with a vast diversity of soil microbes, provides a perfect opportunity for this vital immunological training. It reintroduces your immune system to the ancient microbial allies it evolved alongside.

Here's a tip: Take your shoes off before you go inside your house. Don't track in any chemicals from the garden, road or other pollutants and toxins that contribute to polluted indoor air already inside.

Because here's the uncomfortable truth about your indoor environment: that "new furniture/carpet smell" isn't freshness. It's volatile organic compounds (VOCs) from flame retardants and formaldehyde-based adhesives entering your bloodstream with every breath. Endocrine-disrupting chemicals leach from plastics and cleaning products. Most of us live in an indoor chemical soup linked to respiratory issues and fertility disruption. Add screens that hijack your circadian rhythm and your lounge chairs that slowly destroy your metabolism, and you've got a set up for inflammation and chronic disease.

4. Cooling the Smoldering Fires of Inflammation

> **Watercooler Fact:**
>
> **Cortisol Reset**
> Twenty minutes outdoors, **3x per week**, lowers cortisol by 21%.

Chronic, low-grade inflammation is like a slow-burning fire in the body, fueling conditions from heart disease and diabetes to arthritis and dementia. Fortunately, gardening can help cool it down.

How? By giving your immune system a steady diet of healthy microbial exposure, through the light physical activity that naturally comes with planting and weeding, and through the stress relief that lowers cortisol when you spend time outdoors.

> **Watercooler Fact:**
>
> **Sunlight Is a Vasodilator**
> Thirty minutes of sunlight dilates arteries enough to lower BP by ~5 points.

Research shows that people who garden or spend time in green spaces have lower levels of inflammatory markers such as C-reactive protein (CRP), TNF-α, and IL-6. Caring for your plants is also helping your body turn down inflammation and build resilience for the long run.

5. A Workout for Your Mind and Body

Gardening does not just grow plants; it changes your brain. The simple, repetitive actions of weeding, watering, or planting quiet 'the Narrator of me,' easing rumination and worry. Attention Restoration Theory explains why: your directed focus can rest while your senses engage in soft fascination. Watching a leaf flutter or a ladybug lift off helps restore mental clarity, focus and resilience.

At the same time, gardening is a workout for your brain. Planning what to plant, solving pest problems, and remembering last year's seeding schedules are all complex executive tasks. Research shows that lifelong gardeners have up to a 37 percent lower risk of developing dementia compared to non-gardeners, quite possibly thanks to this continual cognitive challenge.

When you give even part of your seven percent to cultivating a garden, you are not just tending soil or vegetables. You are cultivating clarity, resilience, and a renewed sense of purpose which is medicine for both the brain and the body.

6. Functional Fitness That Feels Like Play

Not everyone loves a formal gym workout. But gardening is an exercise that doesn't feel like exercise. It involves a surprising amount of functional, whole-body physical activity.

Digging: Pushing a shovel into soil and turning it over is a powerful full-body movement. It starts with your legs, which create the leverage you need to move soil. Your core, including the deep transverse abdominis, fires to stabilize your spine. Your back, shoulders, and arms then work together to lift and guide each shovelful.

Weeding: Spending time in a deep squat while weeding is a fantastic functional exercise for improving hip and ankle mobility, often severely limited by our chair-bound lives. Squatting to weed lengthens tight hip flexors and strengthens the glutes and quadriceps through a full range of motion.

Carrying: Hauling bags of compost or full watering cans is a form of farmer's carry, a classic functional strength exercise. It builds tremendous grip strength, challenges your core stability, and improves your overall ability to safely move heavy, awkward objects in the real world.

Gardening beautifully integrates many of the Outdoor Rx principles you've already explored. It's a natural opportunity for joyful, purposeful movement.

7. Flavor and Nutrition You Can't Buy

There's no comparison between a just-picked tomato still warm from the sun and one shipped across the country or from out of the country. That's true for both flavor and nutrition. From the moment a tomato is harvested, its vitamins and phytonutrients begin to erode. Harvesting a tomato when it's fully ripe locks in up to 40% more vitamin C and far higher levels of protective flavonoids than store-bought produce can deliver.

Your senses know when something fresh is good for you. The peppery perfume of basil leaves and flowers, the juicy pop of a sugar pea pod, the snap of a Blue Lake string bean: these sounds and smells signal your body and energize your gut for digestion. Timing matters too. Early morning harvests of leafy greens and herbs yield peak flavor when picked early, before the sun evaporates their fragrant oils. Fruits and pods hit their sugar crescendo later in the day.

Best of all, gardening gives you access to flavors and plant medicines you'll never find on most shelves. Bay, lime and sage leaves have anti-inflammatory compounds. Bergamot oranges are rich in natural cholesterol-lowering agents. Purple eggplants and grapes are dense with resveratrol and powerful anthocyanins. When you care for the soil, it gives you back food, culinary medicine and flavor you can't buy.

The central idea of culinary medicine and the combinations mentioned above is that high-quality, delicious food can prevent and control common health conditions (my ChefMD work). One of culinary medicine's core principles is bioavailability, which means making nutrients in food 'body-ready' so you can absorb more of the good stuff.

When you combine some foods (avocado with fresh spinach, or olive oil with tomatoes, or tea with lemon) you can absorb more of the active good-for-you compounds in the plants. How you choose, combine, and cook your food all affect how much your body can actually use.

Advanced Culinary Medicine

- Inflammation Stack: Tomatoes + olive oil + herbs
- Gut Stack: Fermented vegetables + fiber + prebiotics
- Vagal Stack: Omega-3s + magnesium + bitter greens

Simple kitchen techniques can make a big difference. Adding a bit of healthy fat, like avocado or olive oil, to a salad makes the carotenoids in the vegetables more body-ready and helps you absorb these powerful antioxidants. Similarly, pairing tomatoes and broccoli provides stronger protection against cancer than eating either vegetable alone, especially if the tomatoes are cooked. It's a way of creating Mediterranean flavor and good-for-you on your plate, with which the whole meal becomes more powerful, and more delicious, than the sum of its parts.

Gardeners Have the Power

When you garden, you are simultaneously tending your body and soul. You inoculate your immune system with soil's microbial network, you ground your nerves through mindful presence at the weeding row, and you nourish every cell with produce at its nutrient peak.

Each seed you sow and every bite you take reforge the ancient pact between human and earth. In that simple, earthy alchemy, you reclaim resilience, amplify vitality, and reap a harvest of true, lasting health.

The How-To (Your Mission): Cultivating Well-Being, One Seed at a Time

My patient Greg's idea of a backyard garden was a non-starter. It represented everything he feared: uncontrolled nature, bugs, mess, and dirt. His mission couldn't start there. It had to start where he felt safe and in control.

His first step was the smallest imaginable: a single basil seedling in a ceramic pot on his kitchen windowsill. It was a miniature, living world he could manage. This was his bridge. For you, the starting point may differ, but the principle remains the same: start where you are, with what you have.

Even a single plant can shift biology: research shows that tending to potted plants, indoors and outdoors, lowers blood pressure and reduces stress hormones within minutes. You don't just feel better: you actually are biologically better. Even these small shifts, when repeated over years, are linked with longer healthspan and lower all-cause mortality.

Before you buy seeds or seedlings, remember every successful mission starts with a little research. These four steps apply whether you're working with a balcony, a back porch, or a half-acre.

1. *Observe and Assess Your Space.* Match your ambition to your reality. Count the hours of direct sun, measure your space (a windowsill or a quarter-acre?), and be honest about your schedule and energy. Joy can come from a single plant, like Greg's or much more, but a garden can only be truly productive if you can sustain it. Sustainable habits like these are the backbone of longevity: what you can repeat steadily

is what protects you longest. That's the real secret to longevity: sustainable, repeatable habits.
2. *Start Small.* I like easy wins. A single pot of lettuce seedlings or new baby radishes that go from seed to table in 6 weeks can inspire you and feed you more than a much larger garden you can't maintain. Small, easy wins build momentum, and momentum builds consistency. Consistency matters because repeated light-to-moderate activity outdoors, like gardening or tending balcony plants, lowers cardiovascular risk and blood pressure, and improves mood regulation.
3. *Know Your Foundation:* Learn what you're starting with: if it's contaminated soil, replace it. Buy an excellent organic potting mix. Use a $30 soil tester to test your own soil if you're using in-ground soil. Soil testing can tell you about moisture levels, pH balance, and nitrogen content. The best ones can protect you from urban lead contamination, which can accumulate in bones, damage kidneys, hurt developing brains, and accelerate aging. By protecting yourself from these hidden toxins, you are not just avoiding harm; you are actively preserving your healthspan at the cellular level. Safe, healthy soil is the foundation for a longer healthspan.
4. *Treat Seedlings Gently.* Plants you find in nurseries were often raised in the protective confines of greenhouses, and are not ready for the heat of summer, the rains of Spring, or any other season's inflictions. Let them get used to being outside for a few days, gradually increasing the time each day, so they adapt to sun, wind, and temperature swings. The lesson is the same for us: gradual exposure to new stresses builds resilience. This is also how our own nervous systems adapt: slower, steady exposure builds our resilience and enhances repair mechanisms.

Choose Your Gardening Arena: From Windowsill to Backyard

1. Container Gardening: Your Urban & Beginner's Best Friend

Whether you have a windowsill, balcony, or backyard garden, you should know that even a few minutes of daily green time lowers all-cause mortality and greater cognitive resilience in aging.

The Experience: This is the art of curation, of creating miniature, portable ecosystems. Container gardening is an intimate and controlled conversation with nature. It is about the simple, personal pleasure of pulling crisp lettuce leaves from a balcony box for tonight's salad, or the burst of mint you pluck from a small pot to brighten a glass of water.

For those in apartments or with limited outdoor space, it's a declaration that nature doesn't only exist out there in distant parks. It can be a vibrant, life-giving presence right here in your home. For city dwellers especially, this is no small thing: indoor plants and balcony gardens can significantly reduce anxiety and boost executive function.

Containers are the most accessible and flexible entry point into the world of Gardening Rx, offering a contained and manageable way to get your hands dirty.

This was the only logical starting point for Greg. The idea of a sprawling, unpredictable backyard was his nightmare, but a single, clean ceramic pot was something he could understand. It was a miniature world, like the ones he so meticulously built, but with an important difference: this one was alive.

His decision to order a pot, a bag of sterile organic potting mix, and one small basil seedling was a monumental leap. The bagged soil wasn't the threatening, bug-filled dirt he feared; it was a specified material with a list of ingredients. The pot was a clean, defined boundary.

This absolute control was the bridge that allowed him to bypass his anxiety and focus on the act of nurturing. He could apply his meticulous nature not to arranging tiny plastic trees, but to ensuring this single living thing had the right amount of water and light.

Key Techniques
Companion Planting: Nature's Collaborative Design

Think of your garden as a fine-tuned kitchen brigade. Each player, from parsley to peas, has a role in the feast's success. Plant mint, dill, or cosmos among your tomatoes and suddenly your plot hums with life: ladybugs, lacewings, and mason bees (if you're lucky) are all eager to patrol for aphids or pollinate your fruit tree.

Many herbs dissuade predators, and others attract pollinators. For example, dill and fennel aren't just pretty: they lure parasitic wasps that lay eggs in caterpillars before they chow down on your brassicas. Borage and calendula attract bumblebees, ensuring your beans, zucchinis, and squash set fruit with zeal. Mustard greens and sunflowers can act as sacrificial trap crops, diverting pests away from your prize zucchinis.

A well-designed garden is ecological choreography: when every plant plays its part, the whole garden thrives, and your harvest emerges sweeter, healthier, more abundant, and free of synthetic artificial chemical residues.

Get Your Hands In It--Embracing the Core Activities

Once you've chosen your arena, there are two big buckets: the physical acts of tending your garden, and the mindful practices that turn those acts into powerful medicine.

The Physical Act of Gardening
Prepare Your Soil

Healthy soil is the foundation of a healthy garden. For Greg, using a bagged organic potting mix gave him a sense of safety. For you, preparing your soil is your first act of nurturing. In containers, use a high-quality organic potting mix. In new beds, remove existing vegetation, loosen the soil deeply, and incorporate generous amounts of organic matter, such as compost. Feel its texture and smell its rich, earthy aroma.

Direct contact with soil exposes your skin to beneficial microbes, such as Mycobacterium vaccae, which has been shown to act like an antidepressant by boosting serotonin in the brain. The ideal soil will hold its shape when squeezed but crumble easily when gently jostled.

Plant with Presence

This is an act of pure hope. I watched Greg plant his single basil seedling with the same meticulous precision he used on his models. He centered it perfectly, gently firmed the surrounding soil, and gave it its first drink of water. It was a transfer of his skills from a static world to a living one.

When transplanting, handle vegetable seedlings gently and dig a hole twice as wide as the root ball. If you've started your own seeds indoors, remember the crucial step of hardening off. This is the process of gradually acclimating your tender, indoor-grown seedlings to the harsher conditions of the outdoors to prevent transplant shock.

Water Wisely, Deeply, Well

Water is life, but too much or too little can be stressful for plants. Before you water new seedlings, stick your finger an inch or two into the soil. If it's dry, it's time to water.

It's generally better to water deeply and less frequently than to give light daily sprinklings. This encourages plants to grow deep, resilient roots. Aim the water at the base of the plant, not on the foliage: watering in the early morning is often best.

While sprinkler systems are efficient, they're not always effective at getting water to the roots where it's needed. For a truly water-wise approach, soaker hoses or a drip irrigation system are excellent choices. They deliver water slowly and directly to the soil, reducing evaporation and preventing fungal diseases that can result from wet leaves.

Hand watering with a gentle wand can also be a wonderful meditative practice, allowing you to connect with and observe each plant individually.

Weed Mindfully

Weeds will happen. They're nature's opportunists. Instead of seeing weeding as a battle, reframe it as a meditative act of curating your garden space. Remove weeds when they're small, before they have a chance to set seed. Try to get the entire root.

The process of focused, gentle removal can be incredibly satisfying and calming for the mind.

As you become more familiar with your garden, you can learn to see weeds not as enemies, but as indicator plants telling you a story about your soil. For example, the presence of deep-rooted plants like dandelions or thistles often indicates compacted soil. Weeds like purslane and chickweed usually thrive in rich, fertile, well-balanced soil.

Observing your weeds with curiosity shifts a chore into a diagnostic tool, helping you understand what your garden needs to thrive. I've been taught to look at them as pioneer species: tough things that grow in the tiniest of spaces with the least nutrition. Taking them out by hand (pulling the whole root mass out and shaking off the dirt) ensures they won't continue to grow, and it's my preferred way of weeding.

Harvest with Joy and Gratitude

This is the delicious payoff! Pick your produce at its peak ripeness. As you gather your bounty, take a moment to admire its color, shape, and scent. This is the culmination of your care and nature's magic. And there's a medical payoff: diets highest in homegrown produce consistently predict longer life, lower rates of metabolic disease, and higher cognitive performance.

Engage All Your Senses Intentionally

Gardening is a feast for the senses, offering a direct and powerful pathway to the kind of sensory immersion we've explored throughout this book. As you work in your garden, try hard to tune in.

Observe Your Garden Closely and Regularly

Spend a few minutes each day just looking at your garden. This daily check-in naturally deepens your connection with the principles of mindful observation-- a core skill for understanding nature's subtle cues.

Notice new growth, changes in leaf color, and the arrival of flower buds. Watch for beneficial insects like bees and ladybugs, as well as potential pests. This daily check-in is how you learn the language of your plants.

For Greg, his keen eye for detail, once used to spot a misplaced miniature fence post, was now repurposed to notice the first signs of new leaves on his basil plant. He was learning to read a living system.

I highly recommend keeping a simple garden journal as part of this practice. It doesn't have to be elaborate. Note the date of your observation and jot down what you see. "April 15: First two true leaves on the lettuce seedlings." "May 1: Spotted the first bee visiting the borage flowers." "June 10: Harvested the first ripe strawberry!"

This journal becomes a beautiful record of your garden's journey and a valuable tool for learning and planning for future seasons.

Smell: Inhale deeply. What do you smell? Freshly turned earth? The pungent, peppery aroma of tomato leaves on your fingers? The sweet fragrance of blooming flowers or the sharp, clean scent of crushed tarragon? The musky scent of petrichor (the aroma of rain after hitting dry soil)?

Touch: Pay attention to the textures. The cool, crumbly feel of healthy soil. The velvety softness of a lamb's ear leaf, the rough bark of a tree, the smooth skin of a pepper, the warmth of the sun on your back.

Sight: Go beyond a passing glance. Try to see more than two shades of green. Notice the jewel-like colors of a ripe berry or a vibrant flower. Observe the complex, fractal patterns on a fern frond or a leaf. Watch the mesmerizing play of light and shadow as it shifts throughout the day.

Sound: Listen to the garden's subtle soundscape. The buzz of a contented bumblebee, the cheerful song of a bird, the rustle of leaves in a gentle breeze, the satisfying thud of your spade in the earth, the soft splash of water from your watering can.

Taste: This is the ultimate reward. Mindfully savor the explosive sweetness of a sun-warmed strawberry, the crisp, peppery bite of a fresh radish, the complex flavor of an herb picked moments before you eat it. This is a taste of pure life force.

Practice the One-Minute Reset

To prevent your gardening practice from becoming just another rushed chore on your to-do list, it's vital to integrate moments of stillness. Several times during each session, practice this simple, one-minute reset:

Stop. Put down your tools.

Stand or Sit. Find a comfortable position.

Breathe. Take three slow, deep, conscious breaths. Make each exhale a shade longer than the inhale. This anchors awareness in the senses and triggers a rapid parasympathetic shift via the vagus, offering an immediate, portable reset. Inhale through your nose, and let out a long, audible sigh on the exhale.

Notice. As you breathe, notice any tension in your body, perhaps in your jaw, your shoulders or your hands and consciously let it soften. Let your gaze rest gently on one small, beautiful detail: a dewdrop on a leaf, a bug crawling up a stem, the detailed pattern of a flower petal. This simple act shifts you from doing to being, activating your parasympathetic (rest-and-digest) nervous system.

Return. After a minute, gently return to your task, carrying that small moment of peace with you.

This simple practice re-centers you, deepens your appreciation, and moves your gardening from a physical activity into a moving meditation. The practice elevates your 7% from a statistic to a way to engage and improve yourself. And it ensures that the process continues to nurture you, as you nurture your plants.

The Resolution: Greg Builds a Living World

Greg's single basil plant thrived on his kitchen windowsill. The daily ritual of caring for it became a source of calm. The first time he snipped a few leaves to put on his pasta, the burst of fresh, peppery flavor was a revelation. This small success emboldened him. He bought another pot, this time for mint, and then a small rectangular planter for lettuce. His windowsill became a tiny, edible jungle.

The turning point came one afternoon when he was repotting his overgrown basil plant. He accidentally spilled a handful of the dark, fragrant potting mix onto his clean floor. His old impulse would have been a jolt of revulsion and a reach for his vacuum cleaner. This time, he simply looked at it. Without thinking, he kneeled and scooped it up with his bare hands. He felt the cool, crumbly texture against his skin. There was no panic. There was only the soil.

That spring, Greg took his biggest leap. He bought three large containers and placed them on his small, previously empty balcony. He filled them with soil and planted a compact tomato variety, some peppers, and a cascade of strawberries. His sanctuary, once a fortress designed to keep the world out, now had a thriving outpost of the living world reaching into the open air. His blood pressure had come down. He had found a new way to build worlds: not from plastic and paint, but from water, light, and the rich, microbial life he once feared. He was no longer only a collector; he was a gardener.

Helpful Tips and Bonus Info (Nature Notes & Doctor It Up!)

To help you flourish on your gardening journey, here are some extra practical nuggets, key insights, and reliable tips.

Doctor it Up! Healthy, Living Soil: The Foundation of Your Garden's Vitality

If you take away only one core principle from this chapter, let it be this: feed your soil, not your plants. If you consistently nourish your soil with rich compost and diverse organic matter, your soil will provide your plants with a balanced diet of nutrients. In turn, those healthy, vibrant plants will nourish you. Good-quality organic potting mix for containers is a smart investment in your success.

Your garden makes it easier to eat the way your body thrives: colorful plants and fiber in every bite. You need fermented foods for digestive health, high quality protein, and healthy fats like extra virgin olive oil too. Cook to preserve nutrients and follow the seasons when you can. You improve microbial diversity in your gut and through the gut–vagus pathway, a steadier mood, better energy, and sounder sleep.

Nature Note: Share Gardening with Children

If you have young people in your life, invite them into the garden. Give them their own small pot or patch of earth. Choose easy, fast-growing plants like radishes, sunflowers, or sweet peas. Let them get their hands dirty. It teaches them about food, nature's cycles, and patience, and gives them a joyful dose of microbial exposure. Try a bug hunt with a magnifying glass or create seed bombs from clay, compost, and wildflower seeds to toss into neglected areas on your property. The shared memories will be a precious harvest.

Your Outdoor Rx Action Space: Personal Gardening Rx Reflections, Growth Log & Microbial Musings

My Gardening Rx Log & Detailed Field Notes--Tracking My Journey with the Earth

Date: _____ Approximate Time I Spent Actively Engaging in My Garden Today: _____ mins/hours

My Specific Garden Space(s) I Worked In or Connected With Today: (e.g., "My main raised vegetable bed," "The herb pots on my apartment balcony," "Plot #C-7 at the community garden," "My indoor kitchen windowsill garden.") _____

Today's Key Gardening Tasks, Purposeful Activities, and Gentle Intentions: (Be specific. e.g., "Prepared soil in new bed with compost," "Planted six tomato seedlings and companion basil plants," "Spent a meditative 30 minutes mindfully weeding the carrot patch," "Gave all container plants a deep watering," "Harvested a big bowl of salad greens and sun-warmed strawberries," "Simply sat quietly in my garden for 15 minutes after work, just observing.")_____

Vivid Sensory Moments I Consciously Experienced in My Garden Today: (What smells, touches, sights, sounds, or tastes stood out? Be descriptive. e.g., "The pungent smell of tomato leaves on my hands," "The surprisingly soft texture of a new squash leaf," "The jewel-like red of a ripe raspberry," "The sound of bees buzzing in the lavender," "The explosive sweetness of a cherry tomato right off the vine.")

_____

How I Felt While Gardening/How I Feel Now (My Personal "Benefit Check-in"): (Circle words that resonate or write your own. Be honest: some days are more challenging than others, and that's okay!)_____

My Physical State Felt: Energized/Pleasantly Fatigued (the good, tired feeling)/Stretchy & Mobile/Stronger/Grounded & Centered/Invigorated & Refreshed.

My Mental/Emotional State Felt: Calmer & More Peaceful/Focused & Clear-Headed/Accomplished & Proud/Deeply Connected/Purposeful/Happier & Content/Satisfied/Less Chattery/Stress Released/Hopeful & Optimistic/Grateful/Nurtured & Replenished.

Garden Growth Updates/Harvest Notes/Critter Sightings: (What's new or noteworthy? New sprouts? Flowers blooming? Pests or beneficial insects? What did you choose today and what was it like?)_____

Microbial Musings & Reflections on My Deeper Connection

Did I consciously get my hands dirty today and come into direct contact with the soil? How did that real connection feel on a sensory or even emotional level? What sensations or thoughts arose during those moments?_____

What was the most connecting, nurturing, or joy-sparking moment I experienced in my garden today? What specific elements or actions made that moment so special?_____

What is one new thing I learned today through my gardening practice? (Something about a plant, my soil, an insect, or even about my own patience, creativity, or relationship with nature?)

A gentle reflection prompt for ongoing growth: "Thinking about my experience in the garden today, what is one small, intentional thing I can do during my next session to enhance my sensory engagement, deepen my mindful presence, or create an even greater appreciation for the living earth and its incredible microbial communities?"

The Table Is Not the End of the Garden

If you've read this far, you've already had your hands in the dirt.

You've felt what happens when you reconnect with the earth: not in a metaphor, but in biology. The microbes in the soil aren't just good for the plants you grow; they're part of the healing chain that leads, quite literally, from soil to stomach, gut to brain, leaf to longevity.

Now it's time to finish what the garden started. Because just beyond the garden lies another healing frontier: your kitchen. The work you do with soil, sun, and seeds doesn't end at harvest; it continues through what you choose to prepare, how you combine ingredients, and when you eat. To complete the healing loop between land and body, we turn to the power of food, not as lifestyle advice, but as precision intervention. This is where gardening meets gut health, where the table becomes the final phase of the Outdoor Rx.

Greg was not expecting the kitchen to feel like part of the sanctuary he had built outside. The garden had become a place of quiet victories, one sprouting seed, one new leaf, one fewer bug, one pulled weed, one moment of stillness in a life that had known too much noise. But when he stepped inside to the kitchen with his harvest, something shifted: The kitchen felt as if it quietly invited the next step.

Instead of demanding performance or perfection, it offered a chance to translate growth into nourishment, to let what he had tended now tend to him. For someone who had spent years in survival mode, it felt almost intimate. It was the unexpected tenderness of feeding himself with something he had raised from soil.

Just as a neglected garden can rebound with light, water, and care, so can your cells. Plants that survive drought, pests, and wind, somehow still putting out fruit, remind us that our bodies, like theirs, are built to endure and repair. But only if we give them what they need. And food is one of those needs.

Food is information sent to every cell, every time you eat. Food is your fastest-acting, most consistent, and most pleasurable form of daily medicine.

Food works fast because it speaks the body's native language. Every bite is information, sending chemical signals that shift hormones, metabolism, immunity, and mood within minutes. But there's something more subtle happening too, which isn't captured by markers or molecules.

When the food comes from your own hands, you're proving that care matters. The simple acts of choosing, preparing, cooking, and tasting can lower stress chemistry, steady blood sugar, and soften the edges of anxiety.

I taught Greg to tear his basil leaves by hand, releasing their aroma, and drop them on the hot pasta. He drizzled the dish with extra virgin olive oil, added a pinch of salt, and tasted. The flavor was so much brighter than anything from a jar.

And this is the part most people miss: the kitchen is not the opposite of the garden. It is the continuation of it, a place where what has been grown becomes flavor, and flavor becomes healing.

The Soil Starts the Therapy; the Kitchen Completes It

Here's how it works in practice.

The same radish you pulled from the soil for its crisp spice also contains sulforaphane, a compound that activates your body's detox and repair genes. That's phase II detoxification via the Nrf2 pathway. And when you drizzle that radish with extra virgin olive oil and lemon, you dramatically improve the delivery and absorption of the detox compound.

Or take your kale. If you blanch it lightly, finish with garlic and olive oil, and eat it alongside beans or lentils, you've created a three-way defense: anti-inflammatory, blood-sugar stabilizing, and microbiome-feeding.

That's how you build meals that stack function. I call these Food-as-Medicine Micro-doses, because they're tiny, everyday powerful interventions that require no medical prescription.

They are tiny acts with oversized impact. Their effects arrive quickly, and then return hours later when your energy no longer crashes, your mood remains steady, and your body feels the care you've given it.

The secret of culinary medicine is its ability to train your body to resist the Indoor Epidemic. Food carries the instructions your cells need to repair the damage from inflammation, poor gut health, and a depleted nervous system.

Your kitchen isn't just a flavor factory. It's a pharmacy. Simple choices, like cooking tomatoes with olive oil to boost absorption or adding fermented foods to support your microbiome, build daily momentum.

Greg did not need to understand every pathway to feel the shift. As he cooked, he noticed the way his shoulders settled, the way his breathing slowed, and the way the aromas rising from the pan made the room feel warmer. Cooking stopped feeling like a huge chore and began to feel like a practice, a small ritual that reminded his nervous system that he was safe enough to create something. He was grateful for the time to do it.

This kind of quiet, hands-on attention sends a clear signal of safety to the vagus nerve. The senses do the work and are how we experience nature. The smell of basil, the feel of soil, and the steady rhythm of chopping bring you back into your body.

They pull you out of abstract worry and into real presence. This is how the kitchen restores calm and resilience.

That is the quiet genius of culinary medicine. It changes the body before you even take a bite. The simple acts of chopping, stirring, and tasting awaken circuits of presence and pleasure. They draw you out of rumination and back into your senses. In a world that keeps people trapped in their thoughts, a kitchen can become an unexpectedly powerful place to heal.

Culinary medicine can nudge the nervous system toward balance, calm inflammation, and help recharge the microbiome.

Inflammation: The Smoldering Fire You Don't Want to Taste

Low-grade, chronic inflammation is what researchers now call inflammaging. It's the underlying accelerant for most of what we associate with aging: arthritis, heart disease, insulin resistance, dementia, even cancer.

Food can contribute to inflammation or it can fight it. Growing your own food gives you a head start on dousing the fire.

Greg began to notice how the foods he grew carried their own natural defenses into his kitchen. The sharpness of radishes, the strength of garlic and onions, the scent of fresh herbs, and the deep color of ripe berries all offered compounds that steadied inflammation. He did not need a list to understand this. The plants themselves showed their nutrition, their anti-inflammatory power.

Over time, he began to combine foods, not knowing at all what he was doing, but by just combining what he had harvested at the same time. A warm tomato sauce with a drizzle of olive oil and fresh basil left him clearer and calmer. A handful of berries with mint and lime after dinner steadied his energy. A saute of garlic and broccoli or kale at lunch carried him through the afternoon without a crash.

Eat for Your Inner Ecosystem (Gut Microbiome)

If you've ever pulled a radish from the soil and tasted it right there, you've met the microbiome in action.

Our bodies are not machines. They are complex ecosystems. And nowhere is that more true than in the gut. There, trillions of microbes (bacteria, fungi, viruses, and archaea) produce metabolites that affect everything from immune regulation to neurotransmitter production.

His gut felt different now too. The more plants he ate, the steadier and lighter he felt. The garden was working from the inside out.

The gut, the nervous system, and the body's protein-building machinery form a coordinated network I call the Resilience Core. We are not pausing for a protein deep dive, but it more than earns a mention. Protein supports strength, longevity, balance, satiety, and pleasure at the table. These are the everyday benefits that our bodies need, and part of why simple, delicious, high nutrition meals can make such a big difference to your health and healthspan.

You've just learned how to douse the fire of inflammation. Now it's time to nurture the soil.

Garden-to-Gut: Soil Health = Human Health

When you garden without gloves, you're doing more than connecting to nature. You're inoculating yourself with beneficial soil microbes. One species in particular,

Mycobacterium vaccae, has been shown to reduce anxiety, improve emotional resilience, and even support neuroplasticity. But once that soil microbe reaches your skin or lungs, what happens next depends entirely on what you feed it.

Your microbiome eats what you eat. Many microbes thrive when you feed them fiber and other plant compounds. Think of it as an inner garden: more variety in, more life supported.

As Greg cooked and tasted his way through his garden, he found himself drawn to color. Deep reds, bright greens, purples, and golds each offered a different kind of appeal. He learned to mix variety with simple rules, like nearly everything that is green tastes good together, trusting that a colorful plate naturally fed the ecosystem inside him.

He also learned that fermentation extended the life of his harvest and added new layers of benefit. A spoonful of sauerkraut alongside lentils, a splash of kefir in a morning bowl, or a bit of yogurt with greens made him feel nourished in a deeper way.

When to Pick, When to Cook, and When to Let Nature Lead

Gardening teaches patience. Cooking teaches timing. Together, they teach something rarer: the art of knowing when not to intervene.

Just as you don't tug at a carrot before its time, the same is true for harvesting flavor, nutrition, and satisfaction. After years of studying both metabolic timing and culinary science, I've come to believe that when you harvest your food and how you prepare it can be just as important as what you harvest in the first place.

That timing begins not in your kitchen, but under your fingertips in the soil.

The Garden Clock: Timing the Harvest for Nutritional Power

Plants follow a circadian rhythm, just like you do. They synthesize antioxidants during the day, breathe through their pores at night, and release essential oils in response to sunlight. If you want to maximize the nutrition and flavor of what you grow, it helps to follow their biological rhythm.

Morning is ideal for harvesting greens, when they're crisp, hydrated, and cool. Fruits like tomatoes and berries reach peak flavor in the warm afternoon sun. There's a rhythm to the plants, and the gardener learns it over time.

Raw or Cooked? Let the Plant Tell You

Some plants need heat to release their healing powers. Others lose them with heat. Cook tomatoes, carrots, and spinach to amplify antioxidants. Eat radishes, herbs, and citrus raw to preserve vitamin C and aroma. Trust the plant's chemistry.

Re-Training the Tongue: The Forgotten Flavors

Most people have lost contact with bitter, sour, and umami flavors, even though garden-grown foods still carry them in abundance. Ultra-processed foods mute these flavors on purpose, and that has consequences. They help regulate appetite, activate digestion, and keep you grounded.

Greg realized this the first time he tasted a leaf of arugula straight from his garden. He had not tasted that particular sharpness since childhood, when he used to steal leaves from his grandmother's garden. The flavor was unfamiliar and familiar at the same time. It made him slow down. It made him present.

Bitter greens like arugula, radicchio, and dandelion stimulate saliva and bile, which improve fat digestion and nutrient absorption. Umami-rich foods like tomatoes, mushrooms, fermented vegetables, miso, and aged cheese bring depth that increases satisfaction and naturally slows eating. Sour flavors from vinegar, citrus, and fermented pickles brighten the palate and signal microbial richness.

You can begin gently. Add a handful of dandelion greens to a salad. Stir a teaspoon of miso into warm broth made from your carrot tops and leek ends. Pair a sun-warmed cherry tomato with a spoonful of ricotta and a pinch of smoked salt. Invite these flavors back to the table, and notice how cravings shift. What once felt like a need for sugar or salt becomes instead an awakening to the richness already present in real food.

You might find you need fewer artificial flavorings when your garden can give you umami and brightness and depth.

Little Bites, Big Shifts

Culinary medicine doesn't ask for big changes. It asks you to notice: the time of day, the feel of the leaf, the aroma of the herb in your hand. It asks you to choose a raw radish over a beige candy bar, to roast your tomatoes with a little olive oil, to pair bitterness with beauty.

As a doctor, I measure outcomes. But as a ChefMD, I measure joy: bite by bite, harvest by harvest, in a kitchen that listens to the seasons. The garden will show you when. And your body will tell you how.

Doctor It Up! Techniques: Kitchen Pharmacology

You don't need a mortar and pestle. You need a sauté pan, a citrus zester, and a sense of curiosity. Greg learned this quickly.

The first time he cooked with spices, he tossed them straight into the pan. They barely released an aroma. The next time, he warmed a splash of olive oil and then added the spices. The fragrance lifted almost immediately.

He noticed that a squeeze of lemon at the end of cooking woke up the entire dish. He noticed how tearing herbs by hand felt different from cutting them. None of this required a recipe. It only required attention.

From Garden to Table: Completing the Loop

Greg didn't need permission to grow or pick or tear his own basil into a dish he'd made. He needed practice. He needed flavor. He needed to trust that he, as someone who once feared dirt, could become his own best healer.

When you eat for flavor and health like this, you don't just get more years. You get more you. More strength. More calm. More sleep. More laughter.

You become less inflamed and steadier. Harder to knock down. And more joyful to be around.

Your garden taught you that nature heals.

Your kitchen proves it.

You don't need permission to eat this way.

Chapter 7:
Wind Down with Darkness: Your Nightfall Ritual for Deep Rest

You've navigated the demands of the day. Now, as evening descends, a critical transition occurs: guiding your body and mind from bright stimulation into the quiet, calm, and profound darkness of the evening.

This isn't a passive process of running out of energy. It's active, complex, and absolutely vital.

Sleep doesn't just comfort: it recalibrates your brain, mind, and internal systems.

The path to a sharp mind, stable mood, resilient body, and rejuvenating sleep isn't paved with late-night emails, endless screen scrolling, or one last hour of cramming. Consciously managing this nightly shift from light to dark is paramount for your health.

It's the master key that synchronizes your body clock, optimizes your hormones' crucial dance, and releases your brain's most vital maintenance processes.

Our modern world is robbing us of this biological inheritance.

The Why: Why Darkness is Your Brain's Superpower

To understand how sleep shapes our health, we must first explore the key forces that regulate our internal clock and nightly rest. Here are 11 points to know:

> **Watercooler Fact:**
>
> **Cold-Start Clarity**
> Pairing morning light with **1–3 minutes** of 40–50°F (4–10°C) cold exposure boosts alertness and metabolic activation.

1. Your Master Clock and the Power of Contrast

Deep within your brain in the hypothalamus, sits your Master Clock, mentioned in Chapter 1. This powerful internal clock relies on clear environmental cues, called zeitgebers (time-givers), to synchronize your physiology with the planet's 24-hour rotation. By far, the most powerful zeitgeber for humans is the daily cycle of light and darkness.

Your Master Clock is the moon to your body's tides. It pulls your hormones, digestion, and energy up and down in predictable rhythms. These cycles create peaks of alertness and valleys of rest, regulating everything from performance to healing.

> **Watercooler Fact:**
>
> Depression Light Dose
> One hour of early outdoor light reduces depression symptoms by 50%.

Your Master Clock is the moon to your body's tides, but even the moon needs a cue. For your circadian system, that cue is light. The bright, energizing blue-spectrum light of morning pulls your Master Clock to its peak, and tells your body to rise and shine, alive and bright with energy. In the evening, softening light slows things down. Your Master Clock pulls toward rest, guided by the planet's rhythm.

As the sky shifts from blue to amber at dusk, the light's wavelength changes. Longer red and orange wavelengths reach the special light-sensing cells in your retina that act as dusk detectors. Sunset isn't just breathtaking; it's a primal biological signal to your Master Clock that night is falling. Your body begins its natural descent into rest.

The most important information for your Master Clock is contrast. A bright, unambiguous day signal in the early morning pulls the tide of alertness high. An equally clear night signal, true darkness, allows it to ebb into rest. Without this contrast, your Master Clock loses its bearings.

The problem: In our modern world, we rarely experience true darkness. We live in perpetual, artificial twilight, blurring the vital distinction between day and night, and weakening your circadian rhythm, your body's healing and its performance. Constant evening light effectively confuses our Master Clock, leading to chronic misalignment, linked to depression, metabolic dysfunction, immune disease. The moon's ancient, needed pull on your body grows fainter, and we grow sicker.

2. The Biology of Light Sensing: Your Brain's Private Light Meter

Your eyes do much more than form visual images. They are also your brain's primary light meters.

As we discussed in Chapter 1 and mentioned above, those dusk-detecting cells are in your retinas. They signal to the brain's pineal gland to gear up melatonin production. What makes these light-sensing cells unique is that they have a light-sensitive pigment called melanopsin. Think of the light-sensitive pigment as the sensor, and the light-sensing cells as the private data line to your brain's Master Clock.

These cells respond to shorter wavelengths of light, especially the stimulating blue-wavelength light abundant in natural daylight and, unfortunately, emitted heavily by our artificial light sources and screens.

When blue light hits these cells, they send a powerful, non-visual signal directly to your Master Clock, telling it that it is daytime.

Even some individuals who are fully blind and have no conscious light perception can still have their circadian rhythms set by the light–dark cycle, because their light-sensing cells remain functional. This highlights how fundamental and ancient this non-visual light-sensing pathway is. It is a system designed to detect one thing above all else: the presence or absence of daylight.

3. Melatonin: The Hormone of Darkness

Here the biological magic of your evening wind-down begins.

Melatonin is often called the gatekeeper of sleep, the Dracula hormone (because it only comes out in the dark!), or, most accurately, the hormone of darkness, because the absence of light strictly controls its release.

Its gradual rise in your bloodstream as evening progresses is the primary signal to your entire body that nighttime is approaching. Melatonin promotes drowsiness, helps gently lower your core body temperature (which is necessary to initiate sleep), and plays a key role in coordinating overnight repair processes.

> **Watercooler Fact:**
> Melatonin Suppression: Blue light from screens can suppress your natural sleep hormone melatonin by up to 80%.

The critical punchline for our modern lives: Exposure to light in the evening, especially the blue-wavelength light emitted by electronic screens and energy-efficient bulbs, powerfully and directly suppresses your body's natural melatonin production. It also stifles your body's natural sleep signals.

The devices we turn to for relaxation and escape, in fact, physiologically prime us for alertness and insomnia. You know that late-night Netflix binge? That final scroll through social media on your device before bed? Every minute spent basking in the artificial glow of your screens is like a direct signal to your pineal gland: "Party's on! Melatonin production, shut down!"

> **Watercooler Fact:**
>
> **Brain Detox Curfew**
>
> A **90-minute** screen cut-off allows the glymphatic system to clear Alzheimer's-linked proteins during deep sleep.

This is the biological trap my patient, Emily, the perfectionist, fell into every single night. She believed her late-night study sessions, illuminated by the bright glow of her laptop and harsh library lights, were a mark of dedication. In reality, she was performing a nightly chemical experiment on herself that was guaranteed to fail.

As she stared at her screen, she was shutting down her pineal gland's production of melatonin, essentially telling her brain it was the middle of the afternoon. Her inability to fall asleep easily afterward wasn't a personal failing; it was a predictable biological consequence. She was creating her own insomnia.

4. Cortisol's Crucial Evening Dip

Complementing melatonin's rise, as we've explored in Chapter 3, healthy cortisol should naturally decline in the evening, allowing your stress response system to downshift.

Cortisol's evening dip is required for allowing your body and mind to relax and shift into the 'rest-and-digest-and-repair' mode necessary for truly restorative sleep. Suppose your cortisol levels remain elevated in the evening, perhaps due to chronic stress or inappropriate light exposure. In that case, they can directly interfere with your ability to fall asleep and stay asleep.

This is the physiological explanation for Emily's state of feeling wired but tired. Her late-night studying, driven by anxiety about her exams, created a vicious cycle. The stress of the work kept her cortisol high and the light from her screen powerfully suppressed her melatonin.

Her body was receiving two conflicting signals at once: be stressed and alert from the cortisol and light, and be exhausted from a full day of activity. The result was anxious, non-functional exhaustion that made deep sleep impossible.

5. The Phase Response Curve: Your Clock's Sensitive Window

The effect of light on your circadian clock is not just about brightness; it's about timing. Scientists describe this with the phase response curve (PRC), which shows that the same light can shift your clock differently depending on when you see it.

Light exposure in the early evening or during the first half of your biological night creates phase delays. It pushes back your melatonin release and shifts your sleep drive later. Again, that late-night laptop session or endless doom scrolling or Facebook feed check tells your brain it is still daytime, tricking your system into delaying rest.

Over time, this repeated delay creates chronic social jetlag, where your internal clock is out of sync with work, family, or school schedules. The result is more than fatigue: studies link circadian misalignment to higher risks of obesity, diabetes, cardiovascular disease, and even shorter lifespan.

6. The Brain's Nightly 'Brain Flush': How Sleep Cleans House

For decades, we knew sleep was restorative, but the physical mechanism remained a mystery. That changed dramatically with the discovery of the brain's glymphatic system (see Glossary).

> **Watercooler Fact:**
> One Night Impact: Just one night of sleep deprivation causes measurable buildup of Alzheimer's-linked proteins in your brain.

Think of it as your brain's private plumbing network, a sophisticated waste-clearance pathway that runs alongside blood vessels. Its primary job is to flush out the metabolic waste and toxic proteins that collect in the brain during the intense activity of wakefulness.

The process is elegant and efficient. During the day, as your neurons fire, they produce waste products, including toxic proteins like beta-amyloid and tau, both of which are famously associated with Alzheimer's disease.

Then, at night, something remarkable happens. The brain cleans itself! If you let it.

> **Watercooler Fact:**

> **Brain Flush Reminder**
> Your brain clears beta-amyloid, the Alzheimer's toxin, *only* during deep sleep.

But when deep sleep gets disrupted by stress, scattered sleep cycles, or certain sedatives, the brain's cleanup slows. Those harmful proteins stick around. Over time, they clog the system, damage synapses, and drive the kind of cognitive decline that leads to Alzheimer's.

Here's what's normal: we cycle through 4 sleep stages (Transition, Light, Deep, and REM) every 90 minutes. Deep sleep (also called non-REM sleep) occurs in the first half of our sleep time, and mostly in the first one or two cycles.

Why do we get tired in the first place? One idea: adenosine, a brain chemical, accumulates throughout the day, nudging us toward sleep. Another theory suggests that rest clears space for neurons to form new connections.

Recent research points to something even more fundamental. In certain brain cells, oxidative stress accumulates inside mitochondria, the tiny engines that power each cell. As the buildup grows, the mitochondrial system signals for relief: sleep. From this perspective, sleep may have evolved first as a way to repair and reset mitochondria, with all of its other benefits layered on later.

So, fatigue is not a flaw but a safeguard. It is your biology calling for a tune-up of its power plants. Meeting that call with deep, regular, consistent sleep is not indulgence. It is maintenance for the batteries that run your brain.

Your ability to reach and sustain deep, restorative sleep depends in part on your stress thermostat. When the vagus nerve is functioning well, it slows the heart rate, deepens breathing, and prepares the body for deep, slow-wave sleep. When tone is low and the nervous system stays revved, sleep becomes lighter, more fragmented, and harder to maintain.

Practices that build vagal strength during the day, such as time in nature, slow, deliberate breathing, and supportive connection, make it easier for the brain to reach those deep stages at night. In those stages, the glymphatic system clears waste and resets.

Watercooler Fact:

Sleep Collapses with Age
By age 70, people lose **80–90%** of the deep sleep they enjoyed as children.

During deep sleep, your brain cells actually shrink slightly, increasing the space between them by up to 60%. This allows cerebrospinal fluid to wash through the brain, collecting the metabolic debris and flushing it out into the body's lymphatic system for disposal.

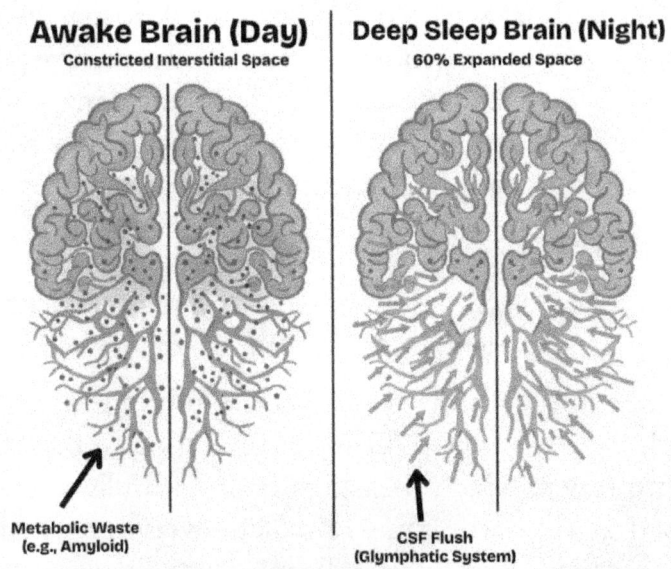

The Brain's Nightly "Brain Flush"

A simple way to remember it: neurons that fire together shower together. Synchronized firing of neurons during deep sleep activates this cleansing shower, which starts within minutes of entering deep sleep.

This nightly brain flush is not optional; it's essential for maintaining brain health. Poor or fragmented sleep compromises this process, leading to toxic protein buildup, which is characteristic of Alzheimer's dementia. And disrupted sleep increases inflammation and oxidative stress, impairs memory consolidation, and impairs neural plasticity. That means more cognitive decline and a higher risk of dementia.

So an impaired glymphatic system has real consequences. Clearance slows, those toxic proteins collect, driving synaptic damage and neuron (aka brain cell) loss. Neuroimaging shows that people with fragmented sleep exhibit shrinkage in memory hubs, such as the entorhinal cortex. Memory shrinkage is a classic early sign of dementia. Without a working glymphatic system, the brain remains smoldering from the day's activities and moves closer toward Alzheimer's and cognitive decline.

7. Sleep Deprivation

Obsessing over hacks while missing the master switches is a common mistake. Sleep is one of those switches.

Every clock in your body syncs when you honor its rhythm. A landmark 17-year study of 45,000 people showed that the Sleep Regularity Index, which measures how faithfully you rise and go to bed at the same times, predicts everything from heart disease to cancer risk to overall mortality. Consistency is not trivial. It is longevity in action.

Research using advanced imaging shows that even one night of missed sleep increases beta-amyloid buildup in the brain, a major risk factor for neurodegeneration. Emily thought all-nighters would help her learn, but each lost hour of deep sleep left her brain unable to clear waste or consolidate memory. The result was brain fog, poor recall, and the exact decline she was trying to avoid.

The Regularity Revolution: Why Consistency Is King

Like many of us, Emily wanted shortcuts. But the right question is not "How many hours did you get?" It is "How consistent are your bed and wake times?" Going to bed and waking up at set times synchronizes your Master Clock, which then drives every cell into rhythm. This is the biology of healthspan: steadier HRV, higher VO_2 max, lower inflammation, and sharper focus.

Morning light and evening darkness are the anchors of this rhythm. Protect them, and you protect the foundation of your longevity.

The quality of your sleep shapes far more than how rested you feel the next day. Circadian rhythms set the heart's timetable, with heart attacks and sudden cardiac deaths peaking in the first three hours after waking, when stress hormones surge. Risk is higher on Mondays and in winter, and it rises further with depression, hostility, and social isolation.

Consistent sleep is protective against heart attacks. The landmark 17-year study of 45,000 people showed those with the most regular sleep schedules had a 34 percent lower risk of heart disease, a 26 percent lower risk of cancer, and a 19 percent reduction in all-cause mortality.

> **Watercooler Fact:**
>
> An estimated 8 to 10 million people in the U.S. use CPAP machines, according to the National Sleep Foundation. Another estimate from The New York Times puts the number at around 8 million. While 39 million U.S. adults have been diagnosed with sleep apnea, many do not use CPAP or may stop using it due to issues with comfort or convenience.

Even with steady routines, disrupted sleep is common, and sleep apnea is a leading culprit. It affects 26 percent of U.S. adults aged 30 to 70, yet only about 5 percent are diagnosed.

Apnea repeatedly interrupts breathing, lowering oxygen, raising blood pressure, and breaking the deep sleep cycles that restore the brain and body. It accelerates cardiovascular aging and increases long-term risk. Treatment can restore restorative sleep and protect both health and longevity.

During deep sleep, the immune system shifts into repair mode, producing infection-fighting cells, repairing tissue, and consolidating immune memory. Poor sleep weakens these defenses, leaving you vulnerable to infections. Good sleep does the opposite: it primes you with the energy and motivation to step outside the next day, where nature further strengthens immune resilience through light, vitamin D and stress relief.

Sleep is also a powerful mood regulator. One night of poor sleep heightens anxiety and irritability, while too little or too much sleep sabotages long-term health. Fewer than seven hours erodes resilience, while more than eight hours increases cardiovascular risk and accelerates cognitive decline by about 12 percent. The sweet spot for most adults is between seven and eight hours.

Finally, sleep and nature work together to keep the brain sharp. Sleep consolidates memory and learning, while time under the open sky restores attention, boosts creativity, and reduces mental fatigue. Together, they create a powerful synergy: quality sleep primes you to engage with the natural world, and time in nature reinforces the rhythms that make quality sleep possible.

8. The Sleep Crisis Across the Lifespan: When We Stop Playing, We Stop Sleeping

When your clock drifts from the 24-hour day, medical problems result. Kids today spend less time outdoors than prisoners in maximum-security facilities. Their days are increasingly structured, scheduled and screen-filled. The result? We're seeing the natural pattern severely disrupted. Delayed sleep shifts bedtime and wake-up until later (teenagers have this a lot). Rising rates of sleep problems in children parallel the broader cultural shift away from unstructured outdoor play.

Adults need our rest. But there are non-24-hour patterns, where the sleep cycle free-runs, sometimes in shift workers. People who get significant jet lag, Seasonal Affective Disorder (SAD, actually a form of depression), who have ADHD, and delayed sleep phases all share the root problem: a misaligned clock.

Night shift work is the modern world's clearest example of circadian disruption. The WHO's IARC classifies it as Group 2A: probably carcinogenic. Light at night suppresses melatonin, a powerful cancer-suppressing agent regulating cell growth and immune function.

There is also serious cardiometabolic damage. Night shift work increases cardiovascular mortality by 27% and metabolic syndrome by 57%, with each five-year stretch adding 7% cardiovascular risk. Consistent sleep and wake times reverse this damage. Highly regular schedules reduce all-cause mortality by 19%: they restore the body's natural circadian rhythm and metabolic function.

The Wisdom of the Nap: Reclaiming Our Natural Rhythm

Here's a truth that our culture desperately needs to remember: napping is not a sign of laziness or weakness. It's a natural, healthy, and beneficial biological rhythm that we've trained ourselves to ignore in favor of caffeine and willpower.

A short nap of 10-30 minutes during this natural dip can dramatically improve alertness, mood, and cognitive performance for the rest of the day. It can also enhance your ability to fall asleep at night, contrary to popular belief, as long as the nap is brief and occurs early enough in the afternoon. The key is to work with your biology rather than against it.

But here's where the connection to nature becomes crucial: the best naps often happen outdoors. There's something about the fresh air, the natural sounds, and the connection to the earth that enhances the restorative power of rest. The afternoon nap in a hammock, the brief rest under a tree during a hike, or even just lying on a blanket in your backyard can be rejuvenating in a way that indoor napping rarely matches.

The person who can take a brief afternoon nap outdoors isn't being lazy. They're being wise. Short naps, especially when aligned with early-morning daylight exposure, can reduce cardiovascular risk, improve metabolic control, and even lengthen telomeres, a biomarker of cellular aging. By stepping outside, you're also counteracting the low Vitamin D, circadian disruption, and metabolic dysfunction tied to spending over 90% of life indoors.

9. The Deception of Sleep Aids

Picture this all-too-common scene: It's 2 a.m. You're tossing and turning, your mind spinning like a hamster wheel. Desperate for relief, you reach for the zolpidem sleeping pills.

But recent data suggest they may nudge up dementia risk in older folks, especially if you're already juggling high blood pressure, diabetes, or a past stroke. One large retrospective cohort even found that higher lifetime use of zolpidem correlates with more Alzheimer's cases later.

The discovery of the glymphatic system and its cleaning abilities lead to a little-known reason sleeping pills may not work as well as you'd like. Common medications like Ambien (zolpidem) may knock you out, but they also suppress norepinephrine. That's the body's chemical signal that drives the nightly brain cleanup. So you do spend more time unconscious, but fewer minutes with the restorative cleansing your brain needs. You get sleep in name, not in function. The brain's nightly dishwasher cycle is switched off.

This may explain why sleeping pill-induced sleep rarely feels refreshing and why long-term use of some older sleep aids has been associated with an increased risk of dementia. They help you check out, but they prevent the cleanup.

Watercooler Fact:

Most over-the-counter (OTC) sleep aids contain either **diphenhydramine** or **doxylamine succinate**, which are sedating antihistamines. Such sleep aids are widely used, especially by students.

Other drugs commonly used also disrupt brain cleaning at night. Benzodiazepines (e.g., diazepam, lorazepam, alprazolam) and anticholinergics (e.g., diphenhydramine, oxybutynin, amitriptyline) impair deep sleep, allowing toxic waste products, like amyloid-β and tau, to accumulate. Long-term use has been shown to impair thinking, memory, and accelerate dementia.

Luckily, orexin receptor antagonists for insomnia exist. A newer class that specifically blocks the wakefulness system, these drugs don't stimulate norepinephrine. They actually suppress the orexin system that promotes wakefulness. Examples include Suvorexant (Belsomra) and Lemborexant (Dayvigo).

Melatonin isn't a sedative, but people use it as one. It's a hormone, and the body's natural night signal. At the right dose (around 0.3–1 mg) and timed correctly, it can actually help deep sleep. But the mega-doses sold in most stores (5–20 mg) often backfire. Large doses desensitize your receptors, change REM sleep balance, and can leave you groggy the next day. In large doses, melatonin weakens the deep sleep your brain depends on to stay sharp.

Watercooler Fact:

CBD is a popular sleep aid, with a significant percentage of users taking it for insomnia, and the CBD industry is large and growing, with a projected market size of over $9 billion in 2024 and an expected increase to over $22 billion by 2030. Approximately 42% of Americans who use CBD do so to help with insomnia.

CBD (Cannabidiol) works differently: by calming anxiety and easing pain, it can help make falling asleep easier. The data about how it affects deep, restorative sleep is mixed. High doses can even be stimulating, and overuse may disrupt sleep quality in ways we don't yet fully understand.

Both melatonin and CBD can help with sleep, but if overused, they put your brain at risk for missing its nightly glymphatic cleansing. Without it, toxins like beta-amyloid build up, increasing long-term dementia risk. Better than supplements is protecting your natural path to fall and stay asleep, and create brain's ultimate detox.

This supports a critical point: not all sleep is created equal. The goal is not just to be unconscious for eight hours. The aim is to achieve naturalistic, functional sleep, rich in the deep, slow-wave stages that enable this vital brain-cleansing process.

Our brains deserve better than quick fixes: they deserve therapies (like unmedicated deep sleep) that clear out neurotoxic proteins at their source. Lean into the simple, time-tested tools you already have: consistent wind-down rituals, nightly screens-off by sunset, and cozy, cool bedrooms that invite true rest.

Sleep optimization is the ultimate Outdoor Rx combo: sunlight, fresh air, soil, and social support. Start your day with the Chapter 1 morning sun protocol to anchor your circadian clock, then weave in a green-exercise break: perhaps a brisk walk through the garden you tend in Chapter 6. Reinforce those rhythms. In the evening, invite a friend to walk at dusk (Chapter 3), using nature's twilight cues to prime your brain for melatonin release. Track your nights with a wearable if you like.

If you monitor your HRV with your wearable, you can peer into your body's stress response and recovery. Follow the impact of your sleep and nature patterns on your health. Lean on these simple, science-backed rituals to remodel sleep from a nightly struggle into wellness writ large.

10. The Modern Saboteurs: Artificial Light and Screens

Our biology is simply no match for the invention of the light bulb and the smartphone.

The widespread, pervasive use of artificial light has changed our environment. Specifically, the blue light emitted so efficiently by LED bulbs, fluorescent lights, and all of our electronic screens is a powerful biological signal. Your brain's light sensors are particularly sensitive to this blue light. When it hits your eyes in the evening, it sends a message to your Master Clock that is loud, clear, and wrong: "It's midday! Stay awake! Do not release melatonin!"

Your circadian clock only responds to darkness if it first gets a strong dose of daylight. Bright morning and daytime light act like charging a solar battery, giving your Master Clock the power to create a clear divide between day and night. Without that contrast, evening darkness loses its signal, and sleep quality suffers.

When you hold your phone inches from your face in a dark room, you're almost shining a personal, miniature sun directly into your brain's light sensors. Because we often hold these devices so close to our faces, the intensity of this light exposure can be incredibly potent, even if the rest of the room is dim. And the effect is not just on our eyes.

Engaging with these bright screens in the crucial 1 to 2 hours before your intended bedtime is the most effective way to hijack your biology, suppress your melatonin, and delay your internal clock, making it much harder to fall asleep and get the deep sleep you need for that vital brain flush.

But here's the deeper story, one that offers even more personal power over your nightly rest: your screen's brightness, how close it is to your face, and how long you're glued to it all play a significant role. One powerful defense you can march out: bright, natural sunlight during the day. The more you soak up during the day, the better your brain fights off the jarring effects of artificial, aka screen light, at night. Your daytime habits literally build a protective shield around your internal clock.

> **Watercooler Fact:**
>
> The average adult spends between **2.5 to 3 hours a day scrolling social media**, though **total screen time can be much higher, with some reports citing as much as 6.5 to over 7 hours a day** across all devices. Social media scrolling alone accounts for an average of about 2 hours and 23 minutes, or approximately 143 minutes, according to recent data.

A second nuance: what you do on your device can pack a bigger punch than its blue light. Playing a video game, scrolling through socials, or texting back and forth with someone keeps your brain buzzing. Those actions hook you, creating neural and mental arousal: not at all what your body wants at bedtime.

Fortunately, your wind-down routine can be a conscious choice for your brain. Maybe skip diving into the new suspenseful Netflix drama and pass on the dense exploration of Norwegian castles. But re-watching a comforting, familiar show or re-reading a familiar book, even on a Kindle or iPad, can have a calming effect. When your brain already knows the outcome, it doesn't have to work nearly as hard, and presto—you can fall asleep more easily.

So, amazingly, it's not all Screen Bad, Sleep Good. For some people, a screen can actually be a tool for better sleep: the right program can kill the rumination circling in your brain. Look for content interesting enough to quiet the voices inside your head, but not so stimulating that it stirs up fears, doubts, excitement, and tomorrow's doings. And when you look for that content, do it outside of bed: your brain should associate your bed with deep, restorative sleep.

The most powerful sleep prescription is the one you write for yourself by listening fiercely to your own body. Your sensitivity to light and screen time is unique. If you fall asleep easily, stay asleep often, and wake up feeling fresh, you're golden. If not, cultivate a wind-down routine that lets you do this.

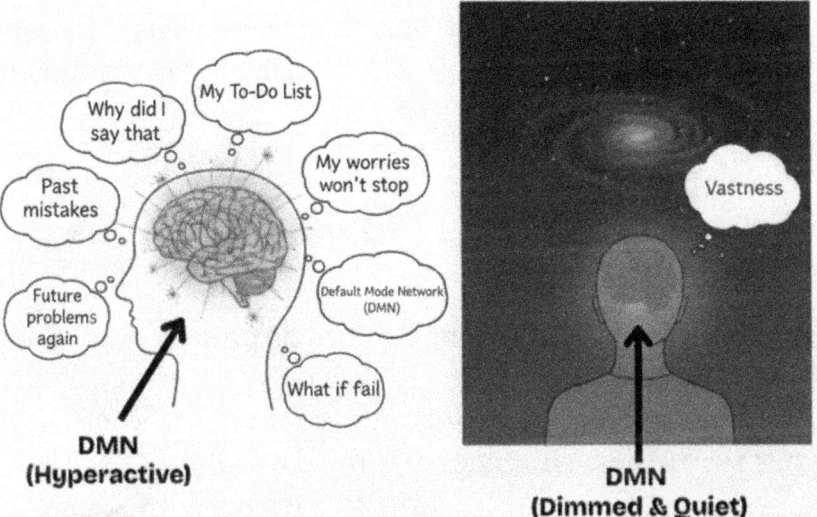

Awe Quiets the "Me" Network

The How-To (Your Mission): The Nightfall Wind-Down Ritual

Darkness is not an absence, but a signal your body depends on. Screens and artificial light can override it, suppressing melatonin and blocking the nightly brain flush that protects memory and long-term health.

For Emily, a driven, pre-med student, the idea of winding down before bed seemed impossible. To her, an unproductive 90 minutes felt like a luxury she could not afford. She eventually learned that this wasn't lost time at all. The critical preparation sharpened her brain, strengthened her memory, and raised her performance the next day.

That is the mission of the wind-down: to create a clear buffer between the overstimulation of the day and the deep rest your biology requires. Think of it as active recovery. What may look like idleness is actually the most important work you do for tomorrow.

Your Six-Step Guide to Better Sleep

1. Crafting Your Pre-Sleep Buffer Zone: The Sacred Landing Strip

Treat the last 60–90 minutes before bed as protected time, and if you can, stretch it to two unhurried hours. It is the bridge between effort and restoration, where your nervous system gets clear cues that the day is done.

It's also a gentle landing strip for your day. Its sole purpose is to consciously and systematically remove sources of harsh stimulation while intentionally introducing calming, soothing cues that signal safety, relaxation, and upcoming rest to your entire nervous system.

Consistency is your friend here. The more regularly you practice your chosen evening wind-down ritual, the more powerfully your body and mind will learn to anticipate and respond to these pre-sleep cues. Over time, the transition into deep, restful sleep will become smoother, easier, and more automatic.

For Emily, this was the first major hurdle. Her journey had to begin with a mindset shift: this wasn't 90 minutes lost from studying; it was a 90-minute investment in making the next day's studying more efficient and effective. She had to learn to see this buffer zone not as an empty void but as an active, vital part of her high-performance strategy.

2. Dim Your Inner World: Create a System of Warm Light

Reclaiming your evenings from artificial light isn't just good sleep hygiene. It's your way of maximizing the restorative power of your 7%. Most of us fritter away those final waking hours bathed in the glow of screens. But you can extract every drop of biological benefit from your time outside the Indoor Epidemic by consciously shifting to darkness (night shift mode on your device helps, but it's incomplete).

The most powerful signal you can send to your brain that the day is ending is to dramatically reduce your exposure to bright, artificial light. This is an important, even critical step in your wind-down ritual.

About 1 to 2 hours before bed, begin reimagining your home from a brightly lit daytime environment into a cozy, warm, and gentle sanctuary.

Kill the Overheads: A Step-by-Step Protocol

- At exactly two hours before bedtime, turn off all overhead lights in your living areas
- If you need task lighting, use only low-wattage table or floor lamps
- In the bathroom, cover or dim harsh vanity lights. Consider installing a separate, dim night light for evening use
- Turn off fluorescent lights completely: these disrupt melatonin production

Switch to Warm, Low-Level Lamps: Your evening should be lit exclusively by low-wattage lamps like table lamps, floor lamps, and bedside lamps. This creates pools of soft, warm light rather than a flood of harsh brightness. Position lamps so they create indirect lighting, with light bouncing off walls or ceilings rather than shining directly into your eyes.

Choose Your Bulbs Wisely: The Technical Details: This is a crucial detail that can make or break your wind-down ritual. When buying light bulbs for your evening lamps, look specifically for those that are labeled soft white or warm white. Even better, look at the color temperature on the packaging, measured in Kelvin (K). Here's your guide:

- 2200K-2700K: Ideal for evening use, giving warm, minimal blue light
- 3000K: Acceptable for early evening but not ideal for the hour before bed
- 3500K and above: Too cool and blue-rich for evening use

For the ultimate in circadian-friendly lighting, consider investing in bulbs specifically designed for evening use. Use amber bulbs that emit virtually no blue light, or even red bulbs for the final hour before sleep.

If you cannot achieve complete darkness for key nighttime tasks, red light is a powerful harm reduction strategy. Your circadian clock is least sensitive to long-wavelength red light (>620 nm). Clinical studies show blue light causes extreme melatonin suppression (7.5 pg/mL), while red light allows recovery to 26.0 pg/mL within two hours, making it substantially less disruptive to sleep onset.

Use dedicated red LED bulbs with peak wavelength 630-670 nm at extremely low intensity, ideally at or below 10 lux at eye level. Place red LED strips at floor level in hallways to minimize direct eye exposure. For therapeutic use, dimmable red lamps can be used 10-30 minutes one to two hours before bedtime to promote relaxation, but turn the light off before sleep.

Embrace the Ambiance --Creating Your Evening Sanctuary: Consider using natural Himalayan salt lamps, which cast a warm, gentle, and calming ambient glow. The soft, flickering, primal light of candles can create a uniquely soothing and tranquil atmosphere, tapping into an ancient human connection to firelight.

If you use candles, please use them with caution: never leave them unattended, keep them away from anything flammable, and be sure to fully extinguish them before you go to sleep.

The aim is to visually, atmospherically, and biologically mimic the gentle, gradual progression of dusk. You're creating a cozy cave, not a bright office.

For Emily, this meant swapping her harsh, blue-white desk lamp for a single, small lamp fitted with a 2200K amber bulb. The change in the quality of light in her study space was the first real signal to her brain that the day was, in fact, ending.

3. Implement a Strict Screen Curfew: Protecting Your Melatonin

This is foundational. It's often the toughest step for most people, but its rewards are immense.

All of your electronic devices including smartphones, tablets, computers, and televisions are potent melatonin-suppressing machines, blasting high-energy blue light directly into your eyes from close range.

The Gold Standard Protocol: The ideal approach is to turn OFF all bright electronic screens at least 60 minutes before bedtime, and ideally 90 to 120 minutes before bedtime. Here's how to implement this systematically:

- Set a daily alarm 90 minutes before bedtime labeled Screen Curfew
- Charge your phone in another room to remove the temptation for just one quick check
- Use a traditional alarm clock instead of your phone
- Inform household members of your screen curfew so they can support you
- Plan your evening activities so you're not scrambling for something to do

Emily's first compromise was to commit to the gold standard for her phone and TV, but she initially felt she had to use her laptop for studying. Her harm-reduction strategy was to wear a pair of dark amber blue-blocking glasses, use an amber desk lamp, and most importantly to do all her reading from her physical textbooks. She used her laptop only for referencing pre-downloaded lecture notes, thus avoiding the temptation of email and the internet.

It was a bridge that allowed her to begin the process.

4. Consciously Shift Your Sensory Input

Your wind-down ritual is an opportunity to curate your entire sensory world for calm. Think about each of your senses and consciously shift their input from stimulating to soothing.

Sound --Creating Your Audio Sanctuary: The auditory environment plays a crucial role in preparing your nervous system for sleep. Here's how to optimize it:

Transition Strategy:

- Hour 2 before bed: Reduce volume of any music, TV, or conversations by half
- Hour 1 before bed: Switch to only soft, instrumental sounds
- Final 30 minutes: Either complete silence or quiet, consistent sounds

Ideal Evening Sounds:

- Nature sounds: Gentle rain, ocean waves, forest ambiance: all tap into our deep evolutionary connection to natural environments
- White or brown noise: Consistent, unvarying background sounds that mask jarring interruptions
- Soft instrumental music: No lyrics, no sudden changes in tempo or volume
- Guided meditations or gentle audiobooks: Choose narrators with calm, soothing voices

Smell --Harnessing the Power of Scent: Scent has a direct pathway to the emotional and memory centers of your brain, making it a powerful tool for creating sleep associations. If you have asthma, chronic lung disease, or allergies, check with your doctor before using diffused essential oils. Some concentrated scents can irritate the airways or trigger symptoms.

Essential Oil Protocol:

- Lavender: The most researched scent for sleep, with proven sedative effects
- Chamomile: Gentle and calming, particularly effective for anxiety-related sleep issues

- Bergamot: Reduces cortisol levels and promotes relaxation
- Sandalwood: Grounding and centering, helps quiet mental chatter
- Cedarwood: Promotes the release of serotonin, which converts to melatonin

Application Methods:

- Diffusers: Add 3-5 drops of essential oil to a water-based diffuser 30 minutes before bed
- Pillow sprays: Light misting of diluted lavender water on pillowcases
- Bath salts: Add a few drops to Epsom salts for evening baths
- Topical application: Dilute properly and apply to pulse points (wrists, temples)

Taste The Evening Beverage Ritual: What you drink in the evening can either support or sabotage your sleep efforts.

Sleep-Supporting Beverages:

- Chamomile tea: Contains apigenin, which binds to benzodiazepine receptors in the brain
- Passionflower tea: Increases GABA levels, promoting relaxation
- Lemon balm tea: Reduces anxiety and promotes calm
- Magnesium-rich drinks: Magnesium glycinate dissolved in warm water can enhance sleep quality
- Warm milk with honey: The tryptophan in milk and the slight blood sugar rise from honey can promote drowsiness

The Timing Protocol:

- Stop all caffeinated drinks by 2 PM: caffeine has a half-life of 6-8 hours
- Limit fluid intake in the final hour before bed to reduce sleep disruptions
- Sip your chosen evening drink slowly as part of your wind-down ritual

Notice that alcohol does not make an appearance! It can be sedating, of course, and may help you fall asleep faster, but it effectively fragments and suppresses deep slow-wave sleep, which you need to clear toxins from your brain.

Part of alcohol's disruption is vagal: alcohol undermines the parasympathetic stability that ushers in deep sleep. Diets high in sugar and ultra-processed foods do the same. An evening ritual that protects your stress thermostat, maybe involving mocktails, teas, or other non-alcoholic, low-sugar drinks, sets up better slow-wave sleep and next-day clarity. A single drink close to bedtime can drop your deep sleep by 20%.

Feel (Touch & Temperature) --Your Physical Comfort Protocol:

The Evening Temperature Transition: Your body's core temperature naturally drops as bedtime approaches. You can enhance this process:

Warm Bath or Shower Protocol: Take a warm (not hot) bath or shower 60-90 minutes before bed. The key is the cooling effect afterward. As your body temperature drops after leaving the warm water, it sends a powerful signal to your brain to sleep.

- Bath Enhancement: Add Epsom salts (magnesium sulfate) to help relax muscles and potentially increase magnesium absorption through the skin
- Shower Alternative: If you don't have a bathtub, a warm shower followed by a cool bedroom works similarly

Creating Tactile Comfort:

- Pajama Protocol: Change into soft, comfortable, and breathable sleepwear made of natural fibers like cotton, bamboo, or linen. This physical act of changing clothes signals to your brain that it's time to transition from day to night.
- Bedding Optimization: Ensure your sheets are clean, comfortable, and made of breathable materials. The physical sensation of sliding into fresh, soft bedding can be a powerful sleep cue.
- Temperature Regulation: Your bedroom should feel slightly cool when you first get into bed. Your body will warm the space naturally.

5. Engage in Genuinely Relaxing, Screen-Free Activities

Watercooler Fact:

Dopamine Without Caffeine

A **10–20 minute** NSDR session increases dopamine by up to **60%**.

This is what your sacred buffer zone is for: activities calming, simple, and free of bright screens. It's not wasted time but the deliberate act of giving your nervous system permission to stand down and prepare for real rest.

One of my patients, Anna, a brilliant lawyer in her late 40s, suffered from chronic insomnia. Her mind was like a courtroom at midnight, filled with endless arguments from worry and regret. Nothing worked until she replaced her late-night phone scrolling with a new ritual: sitting quietly at her east-facing window and watching the moon rise. The slow, predictable arc of the moon gave her anxious mind something vast and steady to anchor to. Within weeks, her sleep deepened and her spirit lifted. What she needed was not a pill, but a dose of the cosmos.

Reading --The Gateway to Mental Calm: Reading a physical book or magazine under a dim, warm-toned lamp is perhaps the most effective and accessible way to wind down. For reading under natural light without the glare or distractions of a traditional screen, an e-reader like a Kindle provides a focused gateway to mental calm and escape, and no blue-light disruption.

Choosing the Right Material:

- *Fiction over non-fiction*: Stories can transport your mind away from daily stresses
- *Avoid highly stimulating content*: Skip thrillers, horror, or anything that might cause emotional arousal
- *Familiar favorites*: Re-reading beloved books can be soothing
- *Poetry or short stories*: These can be perfect for brief reading sessions

The Physical Reading Setup:

- *Lighting*: Use a reading lamp with a warm bulb, positioned so it illuminates the page without shining in your eyes
- *Posture*: Avoid reading lying flat in bed. This can strain your neck and create associations between your bed and wakefulness
- *Location:* Create a cozy reading nook separate from your bed

Gentle Movement --Releasing Physical Tension: Not all movement is stimulating. The right kind of gentle movement can actually prepare your body for sleep.

Restorative Yoga Poses:

- *Child's Pose:* Calms the nervous system and releases tension in the back and hips
- *Legs-Up-The Wall:* Improves circulation and activates the parasympathetic nervous system
- *Gentle spinal twists:* Release tension from the day while lying or sitting
- *Forward folds:* Have a naturally calming effect on the nervous system

Simple Stretching Routine: Create a 10-15 minute routine that targets areas where you hold stress:

- Neck and shoulder rolls to release computer posture tension
- Gentle hip openers to counteract prolonged sitting
- Calf and foot stretches to release the day's accumulated tension

The Worry Dump Technique:

- Set a timer for 10 minutes
- Use your Outdoor Rx journal to write continuously for 10 minutes about everything that's on your mind: worries, to-do items, random thoughts
- Don't edit or organize: just get it all out of your head and onto paper
- When finished, close the journal and mentally leave those concerns on the page

Gratitude Journaling:

- Write 3-5 specific things you were grateful for that day
- Focus on details: not just "my family" but "the way my daughter laughed at my silly joke"
- Include small moments like the taste of your morning coffee or a kind interaction with a stranger
- End with appreciation for your body carrying you through another day

Three Good Things Practice:

- Identify three things that went well during your day
- Write why you think each good thing happened
- Reflect on your role in making these good things occur

Connection and Conversation --The Art of Evening Intimacy: If you live with others, the evening can be a time for meaningful connection that naturally calms the nervous system.

Guidelines for Sleep-Supporting Conversation:

- *Focus on positive or neutral topics*: Save problem-solving discussions for daytime

- *Practice deep listening*: Give your full attention to the other person
- *Share appreciations*: Express gratitude for something your partner or family member did
- *Avoid controversial or stimulating topics*: Politics, work stress, or major life decisions can wait

Family Wind-Down Rituals:

- *Gratitude sharing*: Each person shares one good thing from their day
- *Story time*: Reading together, even with older children, can be deeply bonding
- *Gentle conversation*: Ask open-ended questions about feelings, dreams, or simple observations

6. Creating the Ultimate Sleep Sanctuary: Your Bedroom Environment

Your bedroom environment is the foundation on which all other sleep habits rest. Creating the best sleep sanctuary requires attention to multiple factors that work together to support deep, restorative sleep.

Temperature --The Cool Path to Deep Sleep: Your body's core temperature needs to drop by 2-3 degrees Fahrenheit to initiate and maintain sleep. The brain's thermostat, in the hypothalamus, then can trigger changes that help generate delta waves (the deep, restorative rhythms of sleep). This cooling also boosts melatonin release and allows the glymphatic system to function. This is why the ideal bedroom temperature range is between 60-67°F (15-19°C), with most people sleeping best around 65°F (18°C). Even small deviations outside this range can fragment slow-wave sleep and reduce time spent in REM.

> **Watercooler Fact:**
> **Warm Hands, Faster Sleep**
> Warming your hands and feet helps you fall asleep faster by cooling down your core body temperature.

Darkness --Creating True Night: Achieving true darkness is more challenging than most people realize, but it's critical for maintaining melatonin production throughout the night. Even dim light exposure can suppress melatonin and delay deep sleep onset.

The Complete Darkness Protocol:

- *Blackout curtains or shades*: Invest in high-quality window coverings that block all outside light
- *Light leak inspection:* Walk around your bedroom at night and identify every source of light
- *Electronic device audit*: Cover or remove every LED light, digital clock display, and electronic indicator
- *Door gaps*: Use draft stoppers or weatherstripping to block light from hallways
- *Emergency lighting*: If you need some visibility for safety, use very dim red lights that don't disrupt melatonin

Sound --Creating Acoustic Peace: The ideal sleep environment is completely quiet or filled with consistent, non-varying sounds that mask disruptive noises.

Sound-Masking Strategies:

- *White noise machines*: Steady "shhh" sounds that mask sudden noise spikes
- *Pink noise*: Deeper tones shown to boost slow-wave sleep and memory consolidation
- *Brown noise*: Low rumble that calms the nervous system and rumination
- *Fan noise*: A ceiling or floor fan provides both cooling and background sound masking
- *Nature sounds*: Recordings of rain, waves, or forest soundscape may recall evolutionary relaxation and soothe
- *Earplugs*: High-quality foam or silicone earplugs reduce noise by 25-35 decibels

What to start with? YouTube has many free tracks, and so do many relaxation apps. Experiment and see what your body finds most effective.

Air Quality --The Invisible Factor. The air you breathe while sleeping significantly impacts sleep quality, though it's often overlooked.

Optimizing Bedroom Air Quality:

- *Ventilation*: Ensure adequate fresh air circulation without creating drafts
- *Humidity control:* Maintain humidity between 30-50% for ideal breathing and comfort
- *Air purification*: HEPA air purifiers remove allergens and pollutants that disrupt sleep

- *Plants*: Certain plants, like snake plants or aloe vera, can improve air quality naturally, when loaded in your home in quantity
- *Chemical reduction*: Minimize artificial fragrances, cleaning products, and off-gassing from furniture
- *Shoes at the door*: Reduce the indoor dust and toxin load from outside, including harmful bacteria, asphalt and dirt toxins, synthetic artificial chemicals and lead.

The Psychology of Space --Creating Mental Sanctuary: Your bedroom should be a refuge from the stresses of daily life, dedicated primarily to sleep and intimacy.

Decluttering the Bed and Bedroom for Sleep:

- *Remove work materials:* No laptops, paperwork, or reminders of daily responsibilities
- *Reduce visual clutter*: Keep surfaces clear and storage organized
- *Hidden electronics*: Charge devices outside the bedroom or in closed drawers
- *Calming colors*: Choose soft, muted colors that promote relaxation rather than stimulation

Creating Positive Sleep Associations:

- *Comfortable bedding*: Invest in quality sheets, pillows, and mattresses that make the bed feel like a treat
- *Pleasant scents*: Use subtle, sleep-promoting aromas like lavender if you like
- *Comfort objects*: Soft textures, a special pillow, or meaningful (but not stimulating) objects

- *Ritual space*: Designate areas for wind-down activities like reading or journaling

The Sacred Boundary: Train your brain to associate your bedroom with sleep and rest:

- *No work in bed*: Don't tag your bed as a place of productivity when it should be for rest
- *No eating in bed*: Late-night digestion raises body temperature and can disturb sleep
- *No intense conversations*: Save difficult and emotional conversations for neutral spaces
- *No screen entertainment*: Screens delay melatonin and stimulate your brain; if you use one, dim the light, switch to warm tones from blue, and stick to calm, familiar content.

For Emily, creating this sanctuary was a radical act. It required her to move her desk and laptop out of her bedroom, designating it as a space for rest only. This physical separation created a powerful mental separation, reinforcing the new boundary between her work self and her rest self. That moment reset her trajectory toward understanding that strategic rest is the foundation of sustainable success.

Helpful Tips and Bonus Info

Troubleshooting Common Lighting Challenges

"My partner needs bright light for their evening activities": Use individual task lighting rather than overhead lights, and consider light-blocking glasses for the person who needs to avoid bright light. Create separate zones in your home where one person can have brighter task lighting while the other enjoys dim, warm lighting.

"I live in a small space with limited lighting options": Use lamp shades that direct light downward, and consider light-dimming films for existing fixtures. Even in studio apartments, you can create distinct lighting zones using portable lamps and strategic placement.

"I need to see for safety": Use the minimum light necessary for safety, which is often much less than you think and choose warm-toned options. Motion-sensor night lights with red bulbs can provide safety without disrupting your circadian rhythm.

The Progressive Approach to Screen Curfews

If 90 minutes feels overwhelming, start with just 30 minutes and gradually extend it. The key is consistency, not perfection. Begin by identifying three required elements for your buffer zone: when it starts, how you'll dim your environment, and one calming activity you'll consistently engage in.

Creating Ritual Anchors: Choose specific actions that will become your sleep signals--perhaps changing into comfortable clothes, dimming the lights, and making herbal tea. These ritual anchors become powerful cues that tell your nervous system it's time to begin the wind-down process.

Harm-Reduction Strategies for Screen Use

For those who cannot immediately eliminate all screen use, implement these harm-reduction strategies (understanding these are compromises, not perfect solutions):

Technology Solutions:

- *Blue Light-Filtering Apps*: Use f.lux for computers or enable Night Shift mode on Apple devices. Set these to activate automatically at sunset
- *Screen Brightness*: Manually reduce screen brightness to the lowest possible setting, often much dimmer than you think you need
- *Physical Filters*: Apply blue light-filtering films directly to your screens
- *Distance Matters*: If you must use a screen, position it as far away as possible to reduce light intensity

Blue-Blocking Glasses --What Actually Works:

- Amber or red-tinted lenses that block 90% or more of blue light
- Wraparound style that prevents light from entering around the sides
- Helpful, effective glasses should make white text on a blue background disappear when you look through them

Content Consciousness: Even with protective measures, what you consume matters enormously:

- *Avoid*: Work emails, news, social media, suspenseful shows, financial planning, or anything that triggers stress or strong emotions
- *Choose*: Calm podcasts, meditation apps, e-books on non-backlit e-readers, or gentle music

- *The 30-Minute Rule*: Whatever content you choose, stop consuming it at least 30 minutes before you want to fall asleep

Managing FOMO and Digital Anxiety

Many people struggle with screen curfews because they fear missing something important. Address this by:

- *Setting expectations*: Let people know you're not available by phone after a certain time
- Using Do Not Disturb modes that allow only true emergencies through
- *Morning ritual*: If you're compelled to check your phone first thing, keep it to 2 minutes. Go get your 15 minutes of morning light, then catch up with messages.

Sound Troubleshooting for Better Sleep:

Noisy neighbors or traffic: Use a white-noise machine or a fan to create a consistent masking sound. Brown noise (deeper than white noise) can be effective at masking lower-frequency sounds, such as traffic.

A bed partner with different sleep preferences: Consider separate audio solutions, such as individual sleep headphones or earplugs, for the more sensitive sleeper.

Sudden noises: Address the source when possible (e.g., squeaky floorboards, noisy appliances) or use a consistent background sound to minimize their impact.

Temperature Optimization Strategies:

Programmable thermostat: Set it to begin cooling your bedroom 1-2 hours before bedtime. This allows your body to naturally follow the temperature drop.

Ceiling fans: Create air circulation without the energy cost of air conditioning. Even a small fan can make a room feel 4-6 degrees cooler.

Breathable bedding: Choose natural fibers like cotton, linen, or bamboo that allow heat to escape rather than synthetic materials that trap heat.

Cooling mattress pads: Technology now offers active cooling solutions for hot sleepers, though these can be expensive.

Foot-warming paradox: Warming your hands and feet can help your core temperature drop more quickly, as it increases blood flow to extremities where heat can be released.

Essential Oil Safety and Application:

Safety Note: Always use pure, high-quality essential oils and follow proper dilution guidelines. Some people are sensitive to strong scents, so start with minimal amounts.

Proper Dilution: For topical application, use a carrier oil like jojoba or sweet almond oil. A general rule is 1-2 drops of essential oil per teaspoon of carrier oil.

Quality Matters: Look for oils labeled therapeutic grade, organic, and tested for purity. Avoid synthetics labeled as essential oils.

The Science of Evening Beverages
Avoid These Evening Disruptors:

- *Alcohol:* While it may make you feel drowsy initially, it severely disrupts sleep architecture later in the night, reducing REM sleep and causing frequent awakenings
- *Large amounts of sugar:* Can cause energy spikes and crashes that interfere with sleep
- *Spicy or acidic foods:* Can cause digestive discomfort that keeps you awake

The Resolution: Emily Learns to Sleep Like a Scholar

For weeks, Emily resisted every element of the wind-down protocol. Stopping her studies 90 minutes before bed felt like failure. She compromised, rebelled, and compromised again. She dimmed lights but kept her laptop open and wore blue-blocking glasses while scrolling medical forums until late. She was chasing a hack, and didn't want to give up her edge.

The breakthrough came during finals week. Exhausted, she finally tried the full protocol: screens off 90 minutes before bed, amber lamplight over her anatomy book, a warm bath with Epsom salts, gentle stretches, and a few lines in her gratitude journal. She fell asleep within 15 minutes, slept a solid eight hours, and woke up sharper than she had in months.

Her recall improved. Her anxiety eased. Her test scores jumped. Emily discovered what centuries of scholars had always known: the mind that rests well learns best. Her wind-down wasn't lost study time. The secret weapon made her a better student.

Your Outdoor Rx Action Space: Wind Down with Darkness Sleep Optimization Log

Use your Outdoor Rx notebook notes and reflections to optimize your approach based on what works best for your unique life and schedule.

My Wind Down with Darkness Rx Log--Tracking My Journey to Restorative Sleep

Date: _____ Bedtime Goal: _____ Actual Sleep Time: _____

My Pre-Sleep Buffer Zone (Check all that apply):

Started my wind-down routine _____ minutes before intended sleep

Dimmed/turned off overhead lights

Used warm, low-wattage lamps only

Implemented screen curfew (time: _____)

Changed into comfortable sleep clothes

Engaged in calming activity: _____

My Evening Activities (What helped me wind down?):

Reading (physical book/magazine)

Gentle stretching or yoga

Journaling or gratitude practice

Warm bath or shower

Meditation or breathing exercises

Quiet conversation with family/partner

Listening to calming music or nature sounds

Other: _____

My Sleep Environment Assessment:

Bedroom temperature: _____ °F (Target: 60-67°F)

Darkness level (1-10, 10 being completely dark): _____

Sound level (any disruptive noises?): _____

Air quality (stuffy, fresh, etc.): _____

Sleep Quality Reflection:

How long did it take to fall asleep? _____ minutes

How many times did I wake during the night? _____

How rested do I feel this morning (1-10)? _____

Any dreams I remember? _____

What Worked Well:

What part of my wind-down routine felt most calming?
_____

What made the biggest difference in my sleep quality?
_____

What felt sustainable and enjoyable? _____

What to Adjust:

What challenged me most about my wind-down routine?
_____

What would I like to try differently tomorrow night?
_____

Any barriers I need to problem-solve? _____

Connection to My Daily Rhythm:

Did I get morning sunlight today? (Chapter 1 connection) Yes/No

Did I spend time in nature today? (Connection to other Outdoor Rx practices) _____

How did my daytime activities affect my evening wind-down? _____

My Sleep Intention for Tomorrow: "Tomorrow night, I commit to _____ to support my body's natural transition to restorative sleep."

Remember: Quality sleep isn't a luxury. It's the foundation that makes every other aspect of your health and performance possible. Your commitment to darkness is a commitment to your brain's nightly renewal, your emotional resilience, and your daytime vitality.

Chapter 8: Your 7-Day Outdoor Rx Reset Plan

The Journey from Knowing to Feeling

This chapter is a simple, guided 7-Day Outdoor Rx Immersion and Discovery Week. It's more personal experiment than boot camp, designed to show you how quickly your biology, mind and body can shift when you use your outdoor time well.

You've learned the science behind why nature heals. You understand how light shapes your biology, how movement rewires your brain, and how disconnecting from screens can restore your mental clarity. But it isn't enough to know about it: you have to experience it for it to work.

You understand that just ten to fifteen minutes of morning sunlight can reset your circadian rhythm, that a 20-minute walk can shift your brain chemistry, that stepping away from screens before bed can restore your sleep quality within days.

Your Mission for the Week: The Power of Small Wins

Your mission for the next seven days is to engage with each of the seven core Outdoor Rx Steps. You'll anchor your days with the foundational practices of morning light and evening darkness, and on each day between, you'll explore one additional step as your primary focus.

The guiding philosophy for this week is the Power of Small Wins.

In a culture that often demands all-or-nothing perfection, we'll adopt a different strategy. We'll celebrate the process over perfection. A small win isn't about executing a practice flawlessly for an extended period. It's about the simple, courageous act of showing up for yourself.

A small win is:

- Stepping outside for five minutes of morning sun, even when you're tired and running late
- Putting your phone away 30 to 90 minutes before bed, even if it feels strange and you feel a pull to check it
- Taking a 10-minute walk and intentionally noticing the texture of a single tree's bark
- Choosing the gentle, restorative option on a day when your energy is low, rather than pushing yourself and abandoning the practice

Simple Steps to Implement Outdoor Rx

Limit screens 1-2 hours before bed	Spend 30+ minutes outdoors in evening	Use red/dim lighting after sunset
Put devices away and dim indoor lights	Natural light supports your circadian rhythm	If indoor light needed, choose melatonin-friendly options

Our approach is critical because it builds a positive feedback loop. Each small win generates a feeling of accomplishment and, often, a noticeable, immediate benefit, like a moment of calm, a bit more energy, or a clearer head.

Positive reinforcement builds momentum. It creates an upward spiral of well-being, where the practices become easier and more desirable because you have direct, felt evidence of their value.

This is the antidote to the cycle of guilt and failure that so often accompanies attempts at lifestyle change. This week, we don't fail; we gather data and celebrate every small step forward.

Goals for Your Immersion Week

This guided experiment is designed to achieve four goals.

Experiential Learning & Embodiment: This is about moving from head knowledge to body knowledge. You've read about how morning light can boost your mood or how a walk in the woods can lower your cortisol. The goal this week is to feel it. Pay close attention to the direct feedback your body and mind provide. How does your energy shift? Your muscle tension? Your mental focus? Your overall mood?

Solidifying Your Circadian Anchors: The most fundamental goal is to firmly establish the bookends of your day: Meet the Morning Sun (Chapter 1) and Wind Down with Darkness (Chapter 7). These two practices are your binding daily anchors. They provide the foundational rhythm on which all other well-being practices can be built. If you do nothing else this week, focusing on just these two anchors will create a noticeable shift.

Deep Self-Discovery & Personalization: This week is a data-gathering mission. Your unique biology, lifestyle, and environment mean that some practices will feel more impactful or accessible to you than others. Your goal is to identify which practices feel most needed (addressing your personal pain points like stress, poor sleep, or disconnection), most enjoyable, and most realistic to integrate into your life. This is how you begin to craft your own personalized Outdoor Rx.

Building an Upward Spiral: By intentionally engaging in these practices and noticing their benefits, you build momentum. This week is designed to be the launchpad and offer direct evidence that these micro practices can create lasting change.

Keep these in mind as you move through the week. The goal of this 7-Day Reset is to kickstart a sustainable, health-promoting, positive feedback loop that gives you better focus, energy and healthspan.

Your 7-Day Outdoor Rx Immersion Blueprint

This is your practical guide for the week ahead. It's a flexible blueprint, not a rigid set of rules. Approach it with curiosity and compassion. Adjust it to your energy, your schedule, and your surroundings.

Small changes can bring big wins. Try this in-real-life experiment to see if you can reclaim your energy, clarity, and joy from the grip of the Indoor Epidemic.

Your 7% is calling. It's time to answer.

Preparing for Your Immersion Week

A little preparation can make the difference between a frustrating week and one with a revolutionary and positive impact. Taking 20 minutes before you begin to set yourself up for success is a powerful first step.

Cultivate the Right Mindset: This is the most important preparation. Let go of any pressure. Approach this week with a spirit of open-minded curiosity, gentle exploration, and genuine self-compassion.

You're not being graded. You're a scientist in the laboratory of your own life, gathering data on what nourishes you. Some days and some practices will feel easier or more impactful than others. That's normal. Every experience, whether joyful or challenging, is simply valuable information.

Schedule Your Nature Time with Intention: Look at your calendar for the coming week right now. First, find a realistic time slot for your two Daily Anchors: your morning sun exposure and your evening wind-down. Block these out as you would any important health appointment.

Then, look at the theme for each day and pencil in an up to 60 minute window for that day's practice. Building in this structure provides a framework, but remember to maintain flexibility. If life intervenes, don't abandon the plan. Ask yourself: Can I do a shorter micro-dose? Can I shift the timing?

An initial plan prevents decision fatigue; adaptability prevents overwhelm.

Gather Your Simple Tools: These practices require little special equipment. Your goal is to reduce any friction that might hinder you heading out the door. If you have not been filling out the previous pages at the end of each Chapter, now is your time to write down your plan. You'll need:

- A dedicated notebook and pen for your Action Space reflections. This is key to integrating your experiences.

- Comfortable walking shoes, left in a place where they're easy to grab.
- Appropriate clothing layers for your local weather. A quick check of the forecast each morning can make all the difference.
- A reusable water bottle.
- *Optional*: A small cushion or blanket to sit on (a sit-upon) and a small thermos for bringing warm herbal tea on a cooler day.

Consider creating a designated Outdoor Rx Go-Bag or basket near your door with these items ready.

Communicate Your Intention: If you live with others, briefly let them know that you're doing a 7-day personal experiment for your well-being. You're not asking for permission, but enlisting support.

You might say, "For the next week, I'm trying an experiment that involves getting outside a bit more and dimming the lights earlier in the evening. I'm excited to see how it feels."

This simple act of communication can prevent misunderstandings and invite encouragement from those around you.

The Daily Blueprint

Daily Anchors (Practice Every Day, Days 1-7):

AM Anchor (Meet the Morning Sun): Within 60-90 minutes of waking, get 10-30+ minutes of direct outdoor daylight. No sunglasses. Face the bright sky (but never stare directly at the sun). The goal is to set your master circadian clock, trigger healthy cortisol release, and boost mood-regulating neurotransmitters.

PM Anchor (Wind Down with Darkness): Begin your dedicated wind-down ritual about 90 minutes before your target bedtime. The critical steps are to significantly dim all indoor lights (switching to low-wattage, warm-toned lamps only) and to put away all electronic screens. The goal is to allow for your body's natural melatonin production, calm your nervous system, and prepare for deep, restorative sleep.

Day 1: Setting the Rhythm & Cultivating Baseline Awareness

The Daily Rx Focus: Today is all about establishing your foundation. Your primary mission is to consciously and consistently practice your AM and PM anchors and simply observe how your body and mind respond. There's no pressure to add any other Steps today, unless one particularly appeals to you or fits easily into your schedule. The focus is on the bookends of your day.

Gentle Option: Dedicate your full attention to completing the AM and PM anchors without distraction. Use the Action Space prompts in your journal to thoughtfully record your experience with just these two practices.

Energized Option: During your morning sun exposure, intentionally incorporate 5-10 minutes of Mindful Observation, which is the core of Forest-Bathing Rx (Chapter 3). Choose a single natural object like a plant, a patch of clouds or a puddle and observe it with gentle, sustained curiosity, noticing details you might normally overlook.

Mindful Prompt for Today: Throughout the day, practice periodic 30-second Presence Check-ins. You can set a soft, gentle reminder on your phone or watch for a few times during the day. When it goes off, simply pause. Take one slow, deep breath. Ask yourself: How does my body feel right now (tense, relaxed, energized)? What is my mind state (focused, scattered, calm)? What is my overall mood? The aim is to establish a non-judgmental baseline awareness of your internal patterns before the week's interventions truly begin.

Today's Small Win: Your win today is consistency. Completing both your AM anchor and your PM anchor is a huge victory. You've successfully established the foundation for the entire week.

Day 2: Expand Your Perspective (Sky, Space, and Sea Rx)

The Daily Rx Focus: After establishing your anchors, today's mission is to look up and out, using the principles from Chapter 2. This is a direct counteroffensive against the mental tunnel vision of our screen-bound lives. You'll deliberately engage with the vastness of the sky or a wide-open landscape to quiet your mind and restore a sense of scale.

Gentle Option: Schedule a 15-minute Sky Break. Find a park bench, a patch of grass in your backyard, even a quiet balcony that is comfortable and accessible. Lie back or sit comfortably and simply watch the sky. Observe the color, the clouds, the quality of the light. Let your mind drift. This is a low-effort, high-reward practice in awe.

Energized Option: Embark on a 30-minute Horizon Hunt. Frame your daily walk as a mission to find the best, most expansive view in your neighborhood. Seek out places that offer a long sightline: a hilltop, a bridge over a river, a clearing in the woods, or the end of a pier.

The goal is to experience vastness physically. Bring a film camera along the next time you explore wide open spaces. If you have only a few frames to capture, you might pay closer attention. Pause for the right light, notice the horizon, wait for the wind to pass or to catch the branches or bird you're watching. Looking with intention reveals more than just landscape; it reveals where you stand in it. The photos can become tangible reminders of perspective and wonder.

Mindful Prompt for Today: As you gaze at the sky or the horizon, notice the feeling of your focus shifting from the near field (your phone, your computer screen) to the far field. Can you feel the tiny muscles in your eyes physically relaxing? Notice if your own thoughts and worries seem to shrink compared to the vastness before you.

Today's Small Win: Your win today is the act of consciously shifting your gaze. Every minute you spend looking at the expansive sky instead of a constricting screen is a victory for your nervous system and your perspective.

Day 3: Zoom In & Focus (Mindful Observation)

The Daily Rx Focus: Today, we build on the core skill of Forest-Bathing Rx from Chapter 3: the power of sustained, gentle, and curious attention. You'll dedicate ten to fifteen minutes of uninterrupted time to mindfully observing a single, ordinary natural object. This practice trains your attention muscle and reveals the extraordinary beauty hidden in the mundane.

Gentle Option: Choose a simple natural object, like a smooth stone or a large, simple leaf. Find a comfortable place to sit. For two minutes, explore the object with your senses. Focus on its tactile qualities such as its texture, weight, and temperature. Then, explore its visual qualities (its shape, color variations, and patterns).

Energized Option: Select a more complex object, like a decaying leaf, a pinecone, a wildflower, or a piece of textured bark. Spend 15 minutes performing a slow, mindful contour sketch in your notebook. The goal isn't to create a masterpiece, but to use the act of drawing to force your eye to notice every tiny detail, curve, and imperfection.

Mindful Prompt for Today: During your observation practice, notice when your mind inevitably wanders to thoughts, plans, or judgments. With no self-criticism, gently acknowledge the thought and then patiently return your focus to the object. What new details emerge only after you've been looking for five or even ten minutes? How does your mind feel after this period of focused calm?

Today's Small Win: Your win today is discovery. Notice one small, beautiful detail that you've never seen before. Look for a subtle vein pattern on a leaf or a tiny crystal embedded in a rock. Finding something like that is a complete success.

Day 4: Sensory Soak (Full Sensory Immersion)

The Daily Rx Focus: Today, you'll go deeper into the practice of Forest Bathing Rx, moving from observing a single object to a full sensory immersion in a natural environment. Set aside at least 30-45 minutes (or ideally, 60-90 minutes) for this practice. Choose a place with some trees like a park, a woodland trail, or a botanical garden. The aim is to move extremely slowly, or find a single spot to sit, and consciously engage all of your senses.

Gentle Option: Find a comfortable bench or a spot under a tree. For 30 minutes, simply sit and sequentially rotate your attention through each of your senses. Spend 5-7 minutes just listening to the sounds of the environment. Then, spend 5-7 minutes visually exploring your surroundings without labeling anything. Then, focus on the smells, and finally, the sensations on your skin.

Energized Option: Embark on a full 60 – 90 minute, slow, meandering walk in a wooded area. Leave your phone behind. Pause frequently. Practice some of the specific sensory invitations detailed in Chapter 3. Perhaps bring a small thermos of warm herbal tea to engage your sense of taste.

Mindful Prompt for Today: During your daily life, which of your senses feels the most dominant? Which one feels the most neglected? During your immersion practice today, which sensory invitation felt the most calming, engaging, or surprising to you? Can you feel your nervous system tangibly downshifting with a slower breath, a lower heart rate or a release of muscle tension?

Today's Small Win: Your win today is the feeling of downshifting. The moment you notice your breath has deepened, that your shoulders have dropped, or that your mind has momentarily stopped racing. That's the medicine taking effect. That's a victory.

Day 5: Move with Joy Outside (Mindful Movement)

The Daily Rx Focus: Today's mission is a reset for your brain. That foggy, irritable feeling from too much screen time? It's called Directed Attention Fatigue by neuropsychologists, or mental tunnel vision. Nature is the cure.

Your focus works like a muscle. Use it too long, and it burns out. But step outside to walk a trail, bike under trees and breathe clean air and something shifts. The breeze, the birds, the light on leaves: they capture your attention without demanding it. That's soft fascination and how your brain recovers.

When you're outside like this, it's not because you want to burn calories: it is for focus, for clarity, for a refresh.

Gentle Option: Take a slow, leisurely walk in a park or a quiet neighborhood, focusing on enjoying the scenery and the feeling of your body moving. Or find a quiet spot outdoors to do some gentle Tai Chi, Qigong, or simple stretching.

Energized Option: Choose an activity that gets your heart rate up and feels like play. This could be a brisk hike on a favorite trail, an invigorating bike ride, dancing to music in your backyard, or having an energetic game of fetch with your dog. Choose based on what genuinely sounds fun to you today.

Mindful Prompt for Today: As you move, tune into the relationship between your body and the environment. How does the feeling of your muscles working combine with the feeling of the air on your skin or the sounds of nature around you? Notice how this outdoor movement affects your mood and energy. Can you find moments of genuine fun or flow?

Today's Small Win: Your win today is joy. Finding one moment during your outdoor movement where you genuinely smile, laugh, or feel a sense of playful freedom is a complete and total success.

Day 6: Connect Outdoors (Real Connection)

The Daily Rx Focus: Today, you'll be intentional about sharing time outside with at least one other person, putting the principles of Chapter 5 into practice. This can be a planned event or a spontaneous interaction. The focus is on creating a real, present-moment connection with nature as your supportive backdrop. Stuck inside under fluorescent lights 93% of the time? Could 7% sunshine be your escape?

Gentle Option: Have a casual, five-minute chat with a neighbor on your respective front steps. Call a friend and suggest you both sit outside in your own locations while you talk. Have a simple cup of tea or a picnic with a partner or family member in your backyard.

Energized Option: Be the catalyst for connection. Organize a walk, hike, or bike ride with a friend or a small group. Plan an active game in the park with your family. Or volunteer together at a community garden or a local park cleanup event.

Mindful Prompt for Today: During your interaction, practice being fully present. Put your phone away and out of sight. How does the outdoor setting seem to influence the quality of the conversation or the feeling of connection? Does it feel more relaxed or open than it might indoors? Appreciate the moments of shared laughter, quiet understanding, or easy companionship.

Today's Small Win: Your win today is presence. Have a single conversation, no matter how short, in which you feel you were truly present with the other person. Lose the distraction of your phone. Do that, and it's a powerful victory for your relationship and your well-being.

Day 7: Integrate, Reflect & Plan Your Path Forward

The Daily Rx Focus: Today is about integration. Diligently maintain your AM and PM anchors. Then, revisit your favorite or the most impactful Outdoor Rx practice from the week for one extra dose. The most crucial task for today is to set aside 20-30 minutes of uninterrupted time with your Outdoor Rx notebook for deep reflection and planning.

Gentle/Energized Option: Today, choose which practice from the past week you want to repeat. Choose the one that felt most nourishing, most needed, or most joyful.

Mindful Prompt for Today: As you review your notes from the week, approach your observations and yourself with kindness and curiosity. What patterns emerged? What surprised you? What felt challenging? What practices, insights, or feelings feel most valuable for you to carry forward into your regular life?

Today's Small Win: Your win today is making a plan. Sitting down to thoughtfully reflect on your week and creating a realistic, personalized action plan is the goal of this entire immersion. The step changes a one-week experiment into a lasting lifestyle.

After the Immersion: Your Deep Reflection Guide

You've completed your 7-Day Immersion. You've gathered a week's worth of valuable, personal data on the interplay between nature, your body, and your mind. This is a significant accomplishment worthy of celebration.

The final, crucial step is to distill your experiences into lasting wisdom. Set aside 20 to 30 minutes of quiet, uninterrupted time to work on your Outdoor Rx notebook. Approach this process with the same spirit of kindness and curiosity you brought to the week's practices. There are no right or wrong answers, only your authentic experience.

1. Resonance & Personal Impact

Look back through your daily logs. Go beyond what you think you should have enjoyed and be honest about what you truly did. Which of the steps resonated most deeply with you? Which practices felt most impactful? Was it the sharp mental clarity after a morning sun session, the induced calm of a sensory soak, or the joyful release of an outdoor connection?

Which activities did you genuinely look forward to or want to repeat? Identifying the practices that bring you ease or tangible relief is the first step in building a plan you'll actually stick with.

2. Ease of Integration & Challenges

Which habits slid easily into your life and which hit a wall? That's not a failure. That's intel. Let's use it.

Be specific. Was the challenge logistical (e.g., "Getting to a park for a walk took too much time"), motivational (e.g., "I struggled to get out of bed for the morning sun anchor"), or emotional (e.g., "Sitting still and observing felt agitating at first")?

Understanding the sources of friction and ease isn't a judgment on your willpower; it's critical strategic information for designing a realistic and sustainable plan.

3. Observable Shifts & Tangible Benefits

This is where you become the lead scientist of your own experiment. Review your notes on your physical, mental, and emotional states.

What specific changes, even subtle ones, did you observe? Did your sleep quality improve on the nights you honored your wind-down ritual? Did you notice a difference in your ability to handle stress on the days you practiced mindful observation? Did your energy levels feel more stable? Did you feel more connected to yourself or others?

Look for patterns and correlations between your actions and your outcomes. This direct evidence is the most powerful motivator there is.

4. Key Personal Learnings & Surprises

What were your biggest "aha!" moments from the week? What did you learn about your own patterns, preferences, or your relationship with nature?

Maybe you were surprised by how much you enjoyed a practice about which you were initially skeptical, or discovered that a five-minute micro-dose could have a surprisingly large impact on your day.

Capturing these key insights will help solidify the most important lessons from your immersion week.

Creating Your Personalized Outdoor Rx Action Plan

Based on your reflection, it's time to create your initial action plan. The key here is to resist the urge to do everything all at once. The goal is sustainable integration. You want a lifetime of meaningful 7% moments, not a quick week of Instagramable poses.

Choose just ONE to THREE core practices that feel most valuable, accessible, and sustainable for you to continue as regular habits. You can always add more later.

For each core practice you choose, use the template below to get specific and make a practical plan.

Core Practice #1: _____

WHAT will I do? (e.g., "A 15-minute 'Horizon Hunt' walk to expand my perspective.")_____

WHEN specifically will I do it? (e.g., "Right after I drop the kids off at school, before I check my email.")_____

WHERE specifically? (e.g., "The path around the duck pond at the local park.")_____

HOW OFTEN is realistic for me right now? (e.g., "I will commit to this 3 times per week: Mon, Wed, Fri.")_____

Anticipated BARRIERS? (e.g., "Rainy days, feeling unmotivated, getting a late start.")_____

My Planned SOLUTIONS? (e.g., "For rain, I have a good jacket and will tell myself it's a sensory adventure. For motivation, I'll put my shoes by the door the night before. If I'm late, a 5-minute version is better than none.")_____

Core Practice #2: _____

WHAT will I do? (e.g., "Practice my 90-minute Nightfall Wind-Down Ritual.") _____

WHEN specifically will I do it? (e.g., "Every night, starting at 9:00 p.m.") _____

WHERE specifically? (e.g., "In my living room and bedroom, with all main lights off.") _____

HOW OFTEN is realistic for me right now? (e.g., "I will aim for 7 nights a week, but will be happy with 5 out of 7 to start.") _____

Anticipated BARRIERS? (e.g., "Getting home late from work, social invitations, feeling too tired to do anything but watch TV.") _____

My Planned SOLUTIONS? (e.g., "On late nights, I'll do a shorter 30-minute version. I will let friends know I have a 'no-screens' policy after 9 PM. On tired nights, my go-to will be listening to calming music.") _____

Congratulations. You've completed your immersion and discovery week. You've gathered your personal data, you've reflected on your unique experience, and you've made a thoughtful, realistic plan.

This plan isn't a rigid set of rules to be followed to the letter; it's a living document and a starting point. It's the beginning of a new, more conscious, and more vibrant relationship with the healing power of the world just outside your door.

The journey continues, one small, intentional step at a time.

Chapter 9:
Keeping It Going: Making Your Outdoor Rx Stick

Introduction: From a Great Week to a Better Life

You successfully navigated the 7-Day Reset, experiencing firsthand the clarity of morning sun and the deep peace of an evening without screens. You've identified which of the seven prescriptions resonate most powerfully with you. You may even be feeling your body begin to change, with less tech neck, less dead butt or less fatigue. That initial momentum is precious, like the first powerful surge of a spring thaw, full of energy and possibility. Hold on to that feeling.

Because the Indoor Epidemic is no accident. It's the result of a trillion-dollar attention economy engineered to keep you indoors, glued to screens, and disconnected from your body. Algorithms are designed to hijack dopamine, just as dramatized in popular shows like Severance, where work and life blur into a fluorescent loop. That gravitational pull isn't going away. But now, with Outdoor Rx and your own lived experience of nature's impact, you can restore balance, health, and freedom.

How do you move those positive experiences and well-meaning intentions into consistent, durable, deeply ingrained habits that will reliably support your well-being day after day, week after week, season after season? How do you ensure these practices stick, even when the inevitable complexities and stresses of modern life try to pull you back into old patterns of indoor confinement and digital distraction?

This requires us to look beyond sheer willpower and understand the fundamental mechanics of how our brains actually form routines.

Patient Story: Shonda's Time Famine

To understand the challenge of building lasting habits, meet my patient, Shonda.

At 38, Shonda is a home health nurse and the sole provider for her teenage son, Eli. Her life is a masterclass in relentless demand. Her alarm goes off at 5:15 a.m. She works a long, emotionally taxing shift caring for others, then comes home to a second shift of laundry, cooking, bills, and navigating the complexities of raising a teenage boy on her own.

By the time she finally sits down, she isn't just tired; she's depleted to her core.

For her, going outside doesn't feel like an opportunity; it feels like another demand on her already bankrupt energy account.

"I know we should get outside more," she told me, her voice heavy with fatigue. "Eli used to love his skateboard. But now... it's just easier to let him play his video games. He stays out of trouble, and I can actually hear myself think for a minute. It's not ideal, but it's quiet. I just need quiet."

Shonda and Eli were living in a state of chronic time famine, spending upwards of 10 hours a day indoors, their relationship mediated by the silent glow of screens. She could see the toll it was taking with her exhaustion and Eli's anxiety, but the activation energy required to change felt insurmountable.

Shonda's story is the ultimate case study for the person who has no time or bandwidth for one more thing. Her journey isn't about finding huge, empty blocks of time that don't exist. It's about discovering how to weave tiny, powerful moments of restoration into the fabric of a demanding life, guided by the science of habit formation.

The Science of Habits: Why Trying Harder Fails

Making lasting behavioral change is notoriously difficult.

Our brains are efficient engines, hardwired to conserve energy by running on familiar, automated patterns. Relying solely on sheer willpower or discipline, or waiting for a lightning bolt of motivation, is almost always a recipe for frustration. Willpower is a finite resource, like a muscle that gets fatigued with every decision you make throughout the day. Motivation is an unreliable tide that ebbs and flows.

If we want our Outdoor Rx practices to stick and to become as automatic as brushing our teeth, one powerful way is to leverage the core principles of behavioral science. BJ Fogg has written and taught about this extensively and I recommend his work.

Fogg believes that lasting habits are built on a simple, predictable loop: a Cue (a trigger that initiates the behavior), a Routine (the action itself), and a Reward (the benefit that makes your brain want to do it again). Sustainable change comes from understanding this loop and engineering it to work for you. It's about making your desired habits obvious, attractive, easy, and satisfying. It's not about forcing yourself. It's about designing a system that makes it easy to make the right choice a natural one. This is how you become the architect of your habits, not a victim of them.

Detailed How-To Strategies: Your Architectural Blueprint

These are the eight tools Shonda used to find pockets of restoration in her time-starved world.

1. Anchor to Your Deepest Why

The Science Snapshot: Behavioral medicine consistently shows that intrinsic motivation, or acting in alignment with your core values, helps you stick with healthy habits longer and lowers your stress hormone levels. If you have personal goals powered by meaning (family, purpose, joy) you are likely to have better cardiovascular outcomes (fewer heart attacks) and a lower risk of depression. Your why buffers you against the pull of the Indoor Epidemic, and its screens and sedentary indoor life.

Watercooler Fact:

Heart Attack Timing: Heart attacks peak in the first 3 hours after waking, when stress hormones surge, highlighting our body's daily rhythm.

Your Mission: Before you do anything else, you must unearth and polish your core reasons for undertaking this journey. Vague goals like "I want to be healthier" lack the motivational traction to drive change. You need to get specific and emotional.

For Shonda, her why wasn't about getting more exercise. It was about having enough energy to have a real conversation with Eli, to see him smile, and to model a way of coping with stress that didn't involve screens. It was about connection and presence.

Take the time to refine your why. Frame it not as a task you have to do, but as an expression of who you want to become. Instead of "I have to get morning sun," try "I am the kind of person who prioritizes my energy and clarity so I can be present for my family."

Write your why down. Keep it visible. When motivation dips, reconnect with that core feeling you're aiming for. It's your unshakeable North Star.

2. Master the Micro-Habit (Start Impossibly Small)

The Science Snapshot: Our brains resist big, sudden changes, but they're remarkably good at automating small actions that are repeated consistently.

These micro-habits require virtually no willpower to initiate. Even 1–2 minutes of light outdoor exposure has been shown to improve attention and mood by acting in the brain and lowering activity in the amygdala. Green microbreaks in office workers reduce anxiety and eye strain, and the progression of myopia, in just 40 seconds of viewing natural scenes. Consistency, not duration, is the secret sauce.

Your Mission: Choose your key Outdoor Rx practice and shrink it down until it's almost laughably easy. The primary goal is effortless initiation.

For Shonda, a 20-minute walk felt like an impossible mountain to climb. But her first micro-habit was this: "After I park my car from work, I will put on my sneakers and walk to the end of the block and back." It took less than five minutes. Another was for her morning sun: "While the coffee brews, Eli and I will both stand on our small balcony for one minute."

Your micro-habit for getting morning sun might be: "The moment I get out of bed, I will walk to my largest window and open the curtains fully." Your micro-habit for your evening wind-down might be: "At 9 p.m., I will plug my phone into its charger in the kitchen, not my bedroom." Focus only on repeating this tiny action, day after day. Let the habit and the positive feelings it generates naturally pull you toward longer durations.

3. Optimize Your Habit Stacking

The Science Snapshot: One of the most effective strategies for integrating a new behavior into your life is to stack it on an existing, automatic habit. The established habit acts as a powerful, reliable cue. The formula is simple: after/before [current, automatic habit], I will [new micro-habit].

Linking new outdoor actions to strong existing habits enhances adherence rates by 2–3x. And as little as two minutes outside in the morning light has been shown to stabilize circadian rhythms, improving sleep quality, blood pressure regulation, and daytime energy. That also helps to beat back Indoor Epidemic fatigue.

Your Mission: Become a masterful architect of effective habit stacks. First, identify your most solid anchor habits, things you do every day without fail, like brushing your teeth, pouring your first cup of coffee, or taking off your work shoes. These are your prime real estate for habit stacking. Then, link your new micro-habit directly to it.

Shonda's most powerful habit stack became: "After I take off my nursing scrubs (her cue that the workday was truly over), I will immediately step outside onto the balcony for three minutes of deep breathing before I start making dinner." This tiny ritual became a crucial buffer between her stressful workday and her evening with her son. It was a pivotal transition.

Look at your own routines. Where can you insert a two-minute dose of nature? After I finish the breakfast dishes, I will walk outside to check the mail without my phone. While the water boils for my tea, I will stand at an open window and practice mindful listening.

The key is to make the link immediate and obvious. Create a screen-free sleep zone. Swap your phone for a simple alarm clock and let your bedroom become notification-free and bright light-minimum. Learn to signal your brain when it's time to power down naturally.

In a world always on, choosing darkness and quiet is a radical act of repair. Invite a friend to walk, garden, or just sit outside with you, with your phones off. It doesn't need to be an event. Just a moment of conversation, with no alerts or scrolling to dilute the connection. You'll be surprised how reinforcing, calming, and somehow filling just 10 screen-free minutes can feel. This isn't nostalgia: it's neurobiology and it's the quiet heart of longevity.

4. Schedule & Protect Your Nature Time

The Science Snapshot: Consistently scheduled outdoor time lowers blood pressure, reduces all-cause mortality, and extends healthspan. Treating your 7% outdoors as a real appointment is not indulgence. It's preventive medicine.

Feeling suffocated by 93% screen life? Use The 7% Solution as a pressure-release valve, and guard it like an important health appointment. Consistency is what changes brief outings into cumulative gains in longevity.

Your Mission: Become a fierce guardian of your green time. At the start of each week, look at your calendar and block specific time slots for your Outdoor Rx practices.

Shonda scheduled a 15-minute Decompression Walk for herself on her lunch break three times a week. On Saturdays, she added a 30-minute Park Adventure with her son, Eli. These small, scheduled commitments lowered her stress, steadied her blood pressure, and built the resilience that adds up to longer, healthier years.

Even if you can only block out 10 minutes, do it. This act of scheduling makes it real. And learn to politely but firmly defend this time. If someone tries to schedule over your time, try to offer an alternative time. This is critical self-care, as critical as any other health appointment.

5. Leverage Social Support (Your Nature Tribe)

The Science Snapshot: Social connection itself lowers cortisol, reduces inflammatory markers, and predicts longevity more strongly than exercise alone. Pairing social connection with time outdoors amplifies these effects. When you are both outdoors in daylight and engage in a desired shared activity, you increase oxytocin, balance your circadian rhythm, and lower your risk of high blood pressure. You also, like Shonda, fight anxiety from isolation.

Your Mission: Build your Outdoor Rx support system. This doesn't have to be a large group. For Shonda, her Nature Tribe was just her and Eli. They became partners in their new habits. On days when she was exhausted, Eli would say, "Mom, let's go do our one minute of sun." On days when he wanted to stay inside, she would gently guide him out. They held each other accountable with love and support.

Find your Nature Buddy. It could be a friend, a partner, your teenager, or a neighbor. Make a standing date for a weekly walk. Agree to a simple daily check-in text: "Got my sun in! You?"

The gentle, encouraging accountability makes the journey more fun and far more likely to succeed.

6. Engineer Your Environment (Reduce Friction)

The Science Snapshot: Studies of biophilic design in workplaces show the power of that design. Using plants, natural light, and curved lines to emulate nature lowers employee blood pressure, forces fewer sick days and improves cognitive performance. Screen-saturated, windowless environments are linked to higher rates of myopia, metabolic risk, and shortened healthspan. Progressive workplaces are investing in health architecture for exactly this reason.

7. Audit the Sound Around You

Consider creating a Personal Sound Audit. It's a simple tool that helps you identify the daily noises that drain your energy, spike stress, and disrupt focus without you realizing it. It guides you to track the sounds in your home, workspace, commute, and digital life so you can spot patterns and make small changes that immediately calm your nervous system.

Your Mission: Become a personal choice architect for your Outdoor Rx habits. Make healthy cues obvious and easy. Shonda kept a basketball by the front door, making it natural to grab for a quick five-minute game with Eli instead of defaulting to screens. Keep your walking shoes, a sun hat, and a jacket near the door. Place a nature photo or smooth river stone on your desk. These small signals reinforce consistency, and it's consistency that adds years of healthy life.

At the same time, increase friction for habits you want to reduce. Shonda moved video game controllers into a box in the closet, while the basketball stayed in plain sight.

The simplest and most impactful move for most people is to keep your phone charger outside of the bedroom. This single act of environmental design dramatically increases your chances of honoring your evening wind-down. That daily ritual protects sleep, sharpens cognition, and extends healthspan.

8. Track Your Progress & Benefits

The Science Snapshot: Tracking your behavior increases self-awareness and provides a visual record of your consistency, creating a sense of accomplishment. Self-monitoring of any kind can double your success rate. Even journaling seems to lower anxiety scores and increase resilience against depression. Just reflecting on behavior deliberately remodels those behaviors into long-term health assets. Noticing the positive benefits of a habit acts as a powerful intrinsic reward, strengthening the neural loop in your brain.

Your Mission: Become a mindful observer of your journey. A simple checkmark on a calendar for each day you complete your micro-habit can be incredibly motivating. But go deeper.

The most important thing to track isn't the minutes or the steps, but the feeling. After your practice, take 30 seconds to jot down in your notebook how it made you feel. "Felt calmer after my walk." "Had more patience with Eli after our sun minute."

For Shonda, noticing the direct correlation of a few minutes outside directly translating to more peace inside, was enough internal fuel to keep her going on the hardest days.

9. Master the Art of the Restart (Self-Compassion)

The Science Snapshot: Self-criticism after lapses predicts abandonment, but self-compassion predicts rapid recovery and long-term success. Lapses are not a possibility; they are inevitable. In long-term studies, people who forgive themselves and bounce back quickly after setbacks remain more active and maintain better cardiovascular health over the decades. Perfection is the enemy of consistency, and the Indoor Epidemic feeds on collapse when routines slip. The key is to restart.

Your Mission: Become a master of the compassionate restart. The Never Miss Twice rule is your guide. It is fine to miss one day, because life will always intervene. But commit to never missing two. Even the smallest micro-win the next day resets your rhythm and keeps your healthspan moving forward.

When Shonda missed her walk after a long shift and a crisis with Eli, she did not decide she was a failure. She gave herself grace and began again the next morning. She found wins in the margins: opening the window while making coffee, letting morning light touch her face before her commute, taking calls while walking instead of sitting. Each action was small, but together they built steadiness and resilience.

This is how healthspan grows. Not through overnight life-changing modifications but through repeated recommitments. Each micro-habit interrupts the slow erosion of modern life. Each restart strengthens your biology, sharpens your mind, and compounds into extra years of vitality.

Your Outdoor Rx Action Space: Architecting Your Sustainable Habit System

This is your space to design a personalized system for integrating Outdoor Rx into your life for the long haul. Be thoughtful, honest, and creative.

My Top 1-3 Outdoor Rx Must-Have Habits & My Deepest Why:

List the 1-3 practices you are most committed to making consistent:_____

_____

_____

For EACH, restate your compelling, personal why:

Why #1: _____

Why #2: _____

Why #3: _____

Designing My Micro-Habit & Habit Stack for Each Core Practice:

Core Habit 1: _____

My Micro-Habit (so tiny I can't say no!):

_____

My Habit Stack (After/Before [Existing Habit], I will [My Micro Outdoor Rx Habit]):

_____

Core Habit 2 (if applicable):

_____

My Micro-Habit: _____

My Habit Stack: _____

Engineering My Environment for Success:

What specific, small changes can I make to my physical environment this week to make my chosen habits more obvious and easy?

Change 1: _____

Change 2: _____

My Art of the Restart Compassionate Plan:

When I inevitably miss a session, my compassionate First Aid response to myself will be:
_____

My commitment to Never Miss Twice: The next opportunity after a lapse, my micro-version will be:
_____

Keeping it Fresh & Joyful--One Idea for Novelty This Month:

To prevent my core practices from feeling stale, one new thing I could try is: _____

Chapter 10: Bonus Practices: Extra Ideas for Deepening Your Analog Wellness

Your Personal Medicine Cabinet of Outdoor Rx

You've journeyed through the seven core steps of this book.

You've developed awareness of how the Indoor Epidemic is harming your mental and physical health and what to do to counter its negative impact.

You've learned the seven evidence-based Outdoor Rx practices.

You understand the energy boosting power of morning sun, the expansive calm of the open sky, the deep reset of the forest, the joy of movement, the necessity of real connection, the magic of the garden, and the restorative peace of darkness.

That's a phenomenal achievement.

You've now built the foundation of your Outdoor Rx: light, rhythm, awe, immunity, movement, connection, and recovery. Ahead is a Table of Nature-Based Interventions: advanced tools, each evidence-based and designed to keep your practice fresh, while extending healthspan even further. You do not need them all. Choose the ones that fit, because even a few minutes of the right practice, done consistently, can add years to your life and life to your years.

Quick-Take Table (Top 10 Interventions)

Intervention	Key Longevity Benefits	Notes/Protocol
Sauna Bathing (Dry or Wet)	Up to 40% lower all-cause mortality; 63% lower sudden cardiac death; 77% lower cardiovascular mortality at ~45 minutes weekly.	4–7 sessions/week, 20–30 minutes at ~79°C; both dry and wet saunas effective.
Contrast Therapy (Hot + Cold)	Improves circulation, stress resilience, and immune recovery; combines sauna's mortality benefits with cold immersion's 29% reduction in sickness.	Alternate 12–15 minutes of heat with 2–5 minutes of cold, repeat 2–3 cycles.
Vigorous Intermittent Green Exercise	26–30% lower mortality with only 4.4 minutes/day of vigorous outdoor activity.	Hill sprints, trail stairs, fast cycling; ~30 minutes weekly.
Regular Green Exercise	19–25% lower mortality; every 0.1 increase in local greenness = 4% lower mortality risk.	Brisk walking, cycling, or hiking 150–300 minutes weekly.

Forest Bathing (Shinrin-yoku)	50% increase in NK immune cells lasting 30 days; 12.4% cortisol reduction after a single 2-hour session.	2–6 hours weekly in wooded settings; walking, sitting, or observing.
Cold Water Immersion	29% fewer sick days and reduced inflammation with ~11 minutes weekly.	Cold water ≤15°C; natural immersion or cold showers.
Trail Running	2.5× greater stabilizer muscle use than in road running; improves balance and mental health, and carries green exercise mortality benefits.	2–4 sessions weekly on uneven terrain.
Outdoor Yoga/Tai Chi	50% fewer falls in older adults; cardiovascular and balance improvements.	1–7 sessions/week, 30–90 minutes outdoors.
Horticultural Therapy (Gardening)	Moderate reduction in depression symptoms; improved physical and mental well-being.	60–120 minutes weekly; community or home gardening.

Blue Space Living	Lower all-cause mortality and improved mental health in large international studies.	Residential proximity to lakes, rivers, or coasts (<5 km).

The Seven Steps in this book don't match the Top 10 in the Table, intentionally. I chose them because together they reset your whole system: light, rhythm, awe, immunity, movement, connection, and recovery. These are the fundamentals and the practices anyone can do anywhere, with no gear or special settings required. The table shows plenty of other powerful options (e.g., sauna, surfing, cold immersion), but the Seven Steps are the foundation. They're what make the Outdoor Rx work in real life.

Think of them as a menu. You don't need to try everything. Even a few minutes of the right kind of outdoor time can lower risk, boost resilience, and extend your healthspan.

But the world of nature-based medicine is as vast and varied as nature itself. Now that you've mastered the core curriculum, it's time to explore the electives! These are powerful invitations to explore new pathways for deepening your analog wellness journey. Some dietary supplements show promise, and I actively review the research as it is published, and write about it on drjohnlapuma.com and in the newsletter. For example, early research suggests that low-dose lithium orotate may lengthen the cycle of your biological clock and help stabilize its circadian rhythm. It may also support your brain's nightly glymphatic cleanse, which clears toxins during deep sleep.

Bonus Rx #1: Companion Animal Connection: How Positive Regard Rewires the Brain

The Why: How Positive Regard Rewires the Brain

When our 93% indoor existence is routine, the unconditional love of an animal companion can be a lifeline to nature. For many of us, our most consistent and powerful connection to the non-human world comes through a beloved pet. Interactions with nature don't have to be solitary to be restorative. The key is the quality of attention--is it effortless? Is it completely engaged?

Dogs literally nudge you back into the rhythms of the natural world. Dog walks become micro-doses of green exercise, blending the benefits of fresh air to your immune system with the power of purposeful movement. You get sunlight on your skin for Vitamin D synthesis, an even cadence (with training!) that can calm your vagus nerve, and you get the microbial richness of parks or even neighborhood soil. We evolved to be outdoors, in motion, and in genuine companionship with other creatures.

The simple act of petting a dog or cat and feeling the warmth of their body and the rhythm of their breathing has been shown to trigger a cascade of beneficial neurochemicals. It lowers the stress hormone cortisol while boosting levels of oxytocin.

Companion animals are masters of mindfulness. They live entirely in the present moment, unburdened by past regrets or future anxieties. Their unselfconscious embodiment and keen sensory focus can remarkably pull us out of the chaotic loops of our own thoughts and ground us in the tangible reality of the here and now.

They offer what is so rare in human relationships: non-judgmental acceptance. That's a powerful balm for a stressed and self-critical mind. Animals also give us structure and the need to step outside, breathe deeply, and show up for another living being. Because pets sense our moods instinctively, they cue us to slow down when we're wired, to play when we're stuck, and to be present when all our minds want to do is race ahead.

Companion animals are almost living prescription pads for both our bodies and our spirits, and I recommend everyone have one or know one if you can: it's a personal connection to the natural world.

The How-To: Deepening Your Bond with Your Animal Companion

The Mindful Walk (The Sniffari): Elevate your daily dog walk from a simple chore into a rich, shared sensory adventure.

For at least five minutes of the walk, try hard to perceive the world as your dog does. Let them lead (safely, of course). When they stop to investigate a patch of grass with their incredible nose, stop with them. Be patient. Try to imagine the encyclopedia of smells they're reading. Notice how their ears pivot to catch sounds you might have filtered out. This practice changes a routine task into a meaningful session of both mindfulness and interspecies bonding.

Engaged, Screen-Free Play: When you play with your pet, be fully present. Put your phone away. Get down on the floor. Engage in a game of tug-of-war, roll a ball, or dangle a string. Match their energy. Notice the pure, unadulterated joy they take in the simple physical act of play. That joy is contagious and a powerful antidote to stress, a potent mood booster.

The Co-regulation Break: When you're feeling anxious or overwhelmed, find your pet. Sit quietly with them for a few minutes. Synchronize your breathing to the slow, steady rhythm of their own. Place a hand on their chest and feel their heartbeat. This act of co-regulation with a calm animal can have a remarkably fast and powerful effect on your own nervous system, signaling to your body that it's safe to relax.

Bonus Rx #2: Birding: Your Gateway to Wildness

The Why: Training Your Attention on Winged Messengers

Birding is one of the most accessible and potent forms of nature connection available to us. It's a practice that trains the mind, soothes the spirit, and connects us to the wild, untamed nature that exists everywhere, even in the heart of the most densely populated city.

Birding is a powerful form of mindfulness. It requires you to quiet your internal chatter and extend your senses outward. You learn to listen intently for subtle calls and songs. You train your eye to notice fleeting movements and small details of color and pattern.

The sound of birdsong alone has been shown to improve mental well-being, likely because, from an evolutionary perspective, the sound of non-alarmed birds is a powerful signal of safety to our nervous systems.

The practice of sustained, focused attention on birds is a direct antidote to the fractured, distracted state of our digital lives. It's a workout for your attention circuits. And it can work well for you too: you can stimulate, soothe, and regulate the vagus nerve directly through your voice: humming, singing, chanting, or even gentle gargling engages vagal branches in the throat and larynx.

The How-To: A Beginner's Guide to Birding

The Essential Toolkit: Birding is simple. All you really need is a quiet place and a single bird.

But for most people, it's more fun with two simple tools. First, a field guide. While physical books like the Sibley or National Geographic guides are excellent, the best tool for a beginner is an app like Merlin Bird ID from the Cornell Lab of Ornithology. It can help you identify a bird from a simple description and even identify birds by their song. Second, binoculars. You don't need to spend a fortune; a $100 pair offering 8x magnification is perfect to start.

When and Where to Start: The best time to start learning isn't the busy spring migration, but the quiet of winter. The bare trees make birds easier to spot, and fewer species are around, making identification less overwhelming. Begin close to home. Get to know the birds in your own backyard or a local park. Learn to recognize your local regulars be they juncos, chickadees, cardinals, jays or others, the way you might recognize a new neighbor.

The Practice: Find a comfortable spot and be still. Use your ears first. What do you hear? Try to isolate a single call. Then use your eyes. Scan the trees and bushes for movement. When you spot a bird, try to notice one or two key features before it flies away. Is it small or large? What's the primary color on its head or breast? Then, use your app or guide to try to identify it. The goal isn't to identify every bird, but to become a better observer.

To deepen your listening, borrow a page from the wellness trend (and ancient practice) of sound baths. Traditionally held in groups with instruments such as singing bowls and gongs, the aim is to create a sensation of being enveloped in sound rather than to compose a song. Some research shows sound baths can lower anxiety, ease distress, lift mood, and even slow heart rate, though rigorous scientific examination is in early stages. Sound baths are now available in spas, wellness hotels, and resorts. That acceptance signals something deeper that many of my patients hold too: a craving for healthier, non-pharmaceutical ways to soothe and regulate the nervous system.

Lastly, you can recreate that same enveloping effect outdoors. Instead of letting birdsong or wind fade into the background, treat it as a personal sound bath. Close your eyes (if it's safe) and tune in as if each sound is a distinct note in an unseen orchestra, even if the melody isn't apparent. Let the rhythm of waves, the rustle of leaves, or the hum of insects fill your aural awareness without judgment. That kind of intentional listening steadies attention and quiets mental noise. You may find yourself in a state of calm, clear presence.

Bonus Rx #3: Houseplants: Your Indoor Nature Prescription

The Why: Bringing Nature's Nourishing Power Inside

For many of us, especially those in dense urban environments, our most consistent daily interaction with nature happens indoors. The humble houseplant is far more than a decorative object; it's a living, breathing roommate that can significantly impact your health.

Indoor plants measurably change your physiology and perception. Berman's research suggests this may be due to the fractal patterns in plants, which are more 'semantically simple' for our brains to process, reducing cognitive load. Those patterns also lower heart rate and cortisol level. They also improve your perception of air quality: to improve air quality with household plants, you actually need hundreds in an airtight room.

Caring for a plant with watering, pruning, and observing its growth is a powerful mindfulness practice that creates a sense of purpose and connection that is deeply restorative. In a world of constant digital distraction, tending to a plant is a powerful way to restore your directed attention. That simple act of caring allows your thinking and feeling to shift. Each plant becomes a living reminder of growth, resilience, and connection. The 93%

can feel oppressive, but your 7% in nature is a powerful reset button.

The How-To: Becoming a Conscious Plant Parent

Source Your Plants Ethically: The recent houseplant craze has fueled a dark side: plant poaching. To be a conscious consumer:

Propagate and Share: The best way to grow your collection sustainably is through propagation, or creating new plants from cuttings. Exchange cuttings with friends. Each plant will come with a story.

Buy Local and Do Your Research: Seek local nurseries that grow their own stock, rather than buying from big-box stores whose plants are often sourced from massive, resource-intensive industrial farms.

Avoid Unsustainable Materials: Try to avoid plants grown in peat moss, as its harvesting damages vital wetland ecosystems. Look for alternatives like compost mix or coconut coir.

The Ritual of Care: Change plant care from a chore into a mindful ritual. When you water your plants, be fully present. Notice the weight of the watering can, the sound of the water soaking into the soil. Observe the leaves. Are they healthy? Is there new growth?

This simple, attentive act can be a creative anchor of calm in a busy day. Your indoor plants aren't just décor. They're your daily prescription for calm, connection, and clarity. Keep them close, nurture them thoughtfully, and they'll nourish you right back.

Bonus Rx #4: Immersion, Adventure & Purposeful Healing

The Why: Deeper Doses for a Deeper Reset

While short, frequent doses of nature are the cornerstone of a sustainable practice, an occasional longer immersion can provide a system-wide reset for your nervous system and a powerful shift in perspective. These can range from simple micro-adventures to more structured therapeutic experiences.

The How-To: Choosing Your Level of Immersion

The Backyard Micro-Adventure: You don't need to travel far. If you have a safe, private outdoor space, spend one night sleeping in a tent on your balcony or in your backyard. Seeing the full transition from dusk to night is a powerful way to reset your circadian rhythm.

Adventure Therapy: For those seeking to overcome significant personal challenges, Adventure Therapy offers a structured approach. These professionally guided programs use activities such as hiking, rock climbing, and rafting to build resilience, self-confidence, and teamwork in a natural setting.

Care Farms: A Care Farm is a working farm that provides health, social, or educational care services. It's a powerful, interactive form of Outdoor Rx that combines the benefits of animal connection, the therapeutic act of gardening, the satisfaction of purposeful work, and supportive social connection.

Bonus Rx #5: Nature Art & Creative Observation

The Why: From Passive Onlooker to Active Co-Creator

Engaging with nature through creative expression shifts your relationship with the natural world. Creative nature engagement, such as journaling, gardening, or writing inspired by natural settings, deepens your connection. It moves you from a passive observer into an active participant.

Active participation requires deeper attention than simply observing. This creates a richer, deeper appreciation for often-overlooked beauty and sparks curiosity. The result is often a more joyful immersion in the natural world.

The How-To: Unleashing Your Inner Nature Artist

Nature Mandala Creation: During a walk, mindfully gather interesting found objects such as fallen leaves, small stones, flower petals. Find a clear spot on the ground and arrange your items into a temporary circular pattern. Focus on the textures, shapes, and colors. When you're finished, admire your creation, and then leave it for the elements to disperse.

Intentional Nature Photography: Use your smartphone's camera deliberately to train your eye. Give yourself a focused, 15-

minute assignment: capture only the flight of bees or leaf movement or only interesting textures. The goal isn't to collect snapshots, but to sharpen your ability to see the beauty in the details.

Natural Art: Leaves, twigs and stones are a good start, but natural food dyes from foods can add to your nature art. Smashed berries have vibrant anthocyanins, and dried seed pods can leave long-lasting protein residues. Whole vegetables (like bell peppers and potatoes) and fruits (such as citrus, stone and pom fruit) can be sliced in half and used as natural object prints: they're fun fruit and veggie stamps. Why let go of the creativity we were given?

Doctor It Up! Choosing and Weaving in Your Bonus Practices

You now have a full toolkit of practices. The key is to see this not as another to-do list, but as a toolkit for personalizing and enriching your well-being journey.

Follow Genuine Curiosity: Don't let the 93% indoors drain your vitality. Which practice genuinely sparks your interest? If you crave calm, explore outdoor meditation. If you feel a creative urge, try nature art. If you feel a primal need for direct contact with the earth, make grounding a priority. Let your authentic interests guide you.

Start with Micro-Doses: Today's bonus Rx might be five minutes of mindful birding from your window or 10 minutes of barefoot time on the lawn during your lunch break. Small, accessible additions build momentum and joy.

Indoor Epidemic

Let Sound Lead You: Add a quiet hum of a soft song to your day, whether in the shower, in the car, or in front of your parakeet. Your own voice is a built-in vagal tool, which naturally calms.

Layer and Synergize: Look for powerful combinations. Your mindful walk (Chapter 4) can be done barefoot (Bonus Rx #1) with a friend (Chapter 5). A backyard campout (Bonus Rx #5) is a perfect way to practice your Wind Down with Darkness (Chapter 7).

Bring Nature Indoors: For days when you're truly stuck inside, create an indoor nature connection. For an old-school connection to the outside world without digital distraction, a pocket radio like one from Tivoli Audio offers a kind of sanctuary.

Tending to houseplants is a form of micro-gardening and mindfulness. Playing a high-quality recording of a natural soundscape can lower stress. Maximizing natural light by opening your curtains is a simple but powerful act.

Keep exploring, keep experimenting, and keep finding simple, enjoyable ways to let nature's intelligence and restorative power nurture you.

Your Outdoor Rx Action Space: Exploring Your Bonus Toolkit

This is your space for curious exploration. Look through the menu of Bonus Rx practices in this chapter and reflect on what calls to you. No duty, but consider activating new ways to thrive. You may find here new pathways to joy and well-being.

A reflective prompt for your journal: "Which two or three Bonus Rx practices from this chapter genuinely excite my curiosity or seem to speak to a need I have right now (for creativity, calm, connection, adventure)? For each one I've chosen, what is one tiny, accessible 'micro-dose' version of that practice I could experiment with this week, even within the confines of my daily life and urban environment?"

Conclusion: Seriously, You Belong Outside

We've walked a long path together through these pages. We've explored the science, unpacked the practices, and illuminated the simple yet powerful ways to cure ourselves of the Indoor Epidemic and weave nature's healing essence back into the fabric of your modern life.

You've been given the keys to unlock the door of your indoor confinement.

You've learned about the seven core Prescriptions of Outdoor Rx:

- Starting your day with the biological reveal of Meet the Morning Sun (Chapter 1).
- Restoring your perspective with the expansive power of Sky, Space, and Sea Rx (Chapter 2).
- The deep sensory reset of Forest-Bathing Rx (Chapter 3).
- Finding joy by choosing to Move Like You Mean It (Chapter 4) outdoors.
- Nourishing your fundamental need to Connect For Real (Chapter 5) in natural settings.
- The hands-on magic of Gardening Rx (Chapter 6).
- Honoring your ancient biological rhythm by Winding Down with Darkness (Chapter 7).

Deep sleep triggers your brain's cleanup system, clearing toxins that speed up aging and raise dementia risk. It's how you protect your years.

This framework is your map back to a more vibrant, resilient, and fully human way of being. But reading the map differs from taking the journey. Change happens when the practices become embodied when they are lived.

Nature Connection: Your Prescription for Not Dying Early

Nature connection isn't a luxury-it's a biological necessity. Fortunately, the prescription is short and simple: two to five hours of intentional outdoor time each week.

Lower chronic stress, improved attention, stronger immunity, and deeper social connection all translate into measurable reductions in anxiety, depression, cardiovascular disease, and even dementia. Nature is not just recreation. Preventive medicine slows aging and extends healthspan.

Follow these tools if you want more energy, better focus, and a younger biological clock or to stay sharp, slim down, and slow premature aging. Ninety-three percent of your day may be inside, but are some of your best moments when you finally get out? This isn't just a lifestyle choice; it's medicine your body can't do without.

In the United States, the paradox is striking. We have the hours, as 7 percent of our week spent outdoors but they are mostly incidental and unhelpful biologically. Time spent in parking lots, on commutes, and on sidewalks does not carry the sensory richness your body requires. The task is not to search for more hours. The task is to repurpose the ones you already have.

Jennifer's Homecoming: A Final Story of Rescue

The disconnect from nature is real, but so is our power to reconnect. No one embodies this truth more than my patient Jennifer, who was living the Indoor Epidemic in its most extreme form. She spent more than 22 hours a day inside, and her health was collapsing under the weight of obesity, rising blood sugar, Vitamin D deficiency, fatigue, and joint pain. Once the vivacious life of the party, a woman who gardened and organized salsa nights, she had become a prisoner of her own home.

After the pandemic, a significant weight gain had brought with it more than embarrassment: obesity triggered a cascade of related medical problems. Her internist warned her about rising blood sugar and the onset of Type 2 diabetes. Her blood work showed a low Vitamin D level from lack of sun exposure and no dietary supplementation. Her fatigue and creeping joint pain made movement harder and her world smaller. Each symptom fed the others, creating a cycle that was more medical than cosmetic: the Indoor Epidemic taking root in her biology.

Her rescue mission began with the smallest imaginable step: shifting her secret late-night walk with her dog to twilight. From there came another step, and then a bigger one: standing in the full morning sun for the first time in years. What began as terror became relief. What began as fear became freedom.

This is what recovery looks like: not a single breakthrough, but the gradual return of energy, hope, and connection. Jennifer's turnaround proves that no matter how entrenched your Indoor Epidemic feels, your rescue starts with one small step outside.

Your Personal Nature Prescription

Jennifer's story, like those throughout this book, began with one intentional step. Now it is your turn. Create your own Outdoor Rx plan by asking:

What practice will I commit to? (e.g., 15 minutes of Morning Sun, a weekly horizon walk)

Where will I do it? (backyard, nearby park, balcony)

When will it fit into my daily or weekly rhythm?

How long will I realistically be able to do it? (start with 5–10 minutes; consistency matters most)

With whom will I share it, if anyone? (consider sharing... it helps with establishing your new habits)

The tide of medicine is turning. We're moving away from a model that simply manages disease symptoms and toward one that actively creates the conditions for health and healthspan. Nature-based medicine (the conscious, evidence-based application of nature connection to prevent illness and promote well-being) is at the forefront of this movement.

The Nature-based medicine research base is not complete: as we learn more about exactly what works and how, I want to share it with you at indoorepidemic.com, as well as my curated lists of analog devices that can help and biomarkers to track Outdoor Rx outcomes. We are translating new studies as they come online that help you live with less stress and optimal wellness. I look forward to seeing you there.

You Are Nature: This Is Your Homecoming

Remember this: you are not separate from nature. You never were. I lived through the Indoor Epidemic too: too many days lost under artificial light, hours swallowed by screens, too little sky, and too few water sounds and sights. The cure is not complicated. The science is solid. The actions are simple.

Your body runs on the same elements found in soil and sea. Your biology still depends on the rhythms of light, air, sound, and earth, even if your mind has tuned them out. The shift begins with micro-doses: one dawn walk, one pause among trees, one night of real darkness, one potted herb plant. Each is small, but together they change everything.

I hope you explore the Outdoor Rx possibilities. The practices in these pages are not hacks or trends; they are the original inputs your body evolved to expect. I hope that this book helps you fashion your own prescription.

I'm almost 70, and most mornings, I head outside and choose to start the day with light, air, and movement. It's my way of resisting the pull of the Indoor Epidemic. Wherever you're starting from, you're not alone. There's a world worth walking back into. Your best health, your sharpest mind, your longest, healthiest life awaits.

Glossary

Action Terms for Outside: Your Essential Outdoor Rx Glossary-- a quick field guide to the key scientific concepts and unique terminology you'll encounter. This table provides clear definitions, brief explanations, and a foundation to help you throughout the book.

- **7% Solution**: The core concept that the small percentage of time (typically 7%) that most people spend outdoors can be leveraged intentionally, like medicine, to repurpose scattered outdoor minutes into concentrated healing doses for enhanced longevity and vitality.

- **Attention Restoration Theory (ART)**: A theory proposing that natural environments are uniquely suited to restoring depleted 'directed attention' (focused, effortful concentration, fatigued by demands like screen time) by providing 'soft fascination' that effortlessly captures attention, allowing cognitive resources to rest and recharge.

- **Blue Mind**: A mildly meditative state characterized by calm, peace, unity, and a sense of general happiness and satisfaction, specifically triggered by proximity to water.

- **Circadian Rhythm**: The body's complex internal 24-hour clock, or master operating system. It synchronizes virtually every part of your body's systems including sleep-wake cycles, hormone production, and metabolism with the planet's daily cycle of light and dark.

- **Cortisol**: Often called the hormone of action, a natural rocket fuel released in a healthy morning surge (Cortisol Awakening Response, or CAR) to mobilize energy, sharpen focus, and regulate inflammation. Chronically elevated cortisol, however, caused by unremitting stress, is damaging, disrupting sleep, impairing cognitive function, promoting weight gain, and suppressing immune function.

- **Default Mode Network (DMN)**: The Narrator of me. A network of brain regions most active when the mind is not focused on a specific external task, involved in mind-wandering, daydreaming, and self-referential thought. An overactive DMN is associated with rumination, anxiety, and depression.

- **Dopamine**: A key neuromodulator critical for generating motivation, drive, and controlling working memory (the brain's active mental scratchpad), rather than just being a pleasure molecule.

- **Glymphatic System**: The brain's sophisticated waste-clearance pathway that activates during deep sleep, where brain cells shrink to allow cerebrospinal fluid to flush out metabolic waste and toxic proteins (like beta-amyloid and tau) that collect during wakefulness.

- **Gut Microbiome**: The trillions of microbes living in the gut, on the skin, and in the respiratory tract, fundamental for digesting food, synthesizing vitamins, regulating mood, and training the immune system. Its diversity is critical for overall health and is influenced by environmental exposure.

- **Healthspan**: The years of vibrant, active, and joyful life, distinct from mere lifespan, representing the duration of healthy, functional living.

- **Heart Rate Variability (HRV)**: Found on most smart watches and wearables, HRV is the millisecond-by-millisecond change in the intervals between heartbeats. It is more a measure of stress than of the heart, and its patterns are best viewed as trends. HRV reflects the nervous system's flexibility and resilience. High HRV reflects a strong parasympathetic (i.e., rest-and-digest) system and is desirable, while low HRV suggests stress and difficulty recovering, which is not.

- **Indoor Epidemic**: A modern public health crisis characterized by people spending approximately 93% of their time indoors, leading to physical damage (e.g., Tech Neck, Dead Butt Syndrome), systemic breakdowns (e.g., poor air quality, weakened immune system, disrupted sleep), and deep biological damage (e.g., myopia, accelerated aging, brain shrinkage) due to lack of exposure to natural elements.

- **Inflammation/Inflammaging**: Chronic, low-grade inflammation is a smoldering fire underlying nearly every major modern disease, contributing to tissue damage and accelerating cellular aging by shortening telomeres. Inflammaging specifically refers to this process of accelerated aging driven by chronic inflammation.

- **Intrinsically Photosensitive Retinal Ganglion Cells (ipRGCs)**: Light-sensing cells: specialized photoreceptor cells in the retina (distinct from those used for vision) that act as the brain's light meters. They detect overall brightness and color spectrum, particularly blue and green light, and send signals directly to the SCN (or Master Clock) to regulate circadian rhythms.

- **Natural Killer (NK) Cells**: A vital type of white blood cell that acts as the immune system's elite special forces, tasked with identifying and destroying virally infected cells and nascent tumor cells, crucial for a robust immune response.

- **Neuroplasticity**: The brain's remarkable ability to reorganize itself by forming new neural connections throughout life, which is supported by activities like exercise and learning.

- **Old Friends Hypothesis**: A theory in immunology positing that human immune systems co-evolved with diverse microorganisms from nature, and regular exposure to these old friends is required for proper immune system development, calibration, and tolerance, preventing overreactions like allergies and autoimmune diseases.

- **Oxytocin**: Often called the bonding hormone or cuddle chemical, a powerful neuropeptide released during genuine social connection that promotes feelings of trust, safety, empathy, and generosity, and directly counteracts the physiological effects of cortisol.

- **Phytoncides**: Airborne aromatic compounds produced by trees and plants as part of their natural immune system. When inhaled, these compounds significantly boost human immune function, particularly by increasing the number and activity of Natural Killer (NK) cells.

- **Suprachiasmatic Nucleus (SCN)**: A tiny, powerful cluster of nerve cells in the hypothalamus that functions as the body's central Master Clock, coordinating biological operations and synchronizing peripheral clocks throughout the body based on environmental cues, especially light.

- **Telomeres**: Regions of repetitive DNA sequences at the end of a chromosome (a sort of shoelace tip on a shoelace) that protects the chromosome from damage and from scrambling genetic information. With aging and stress, telomeres wear down and can eventually kill cells.

- **Vagus Nerve**: The body's longest parasympathetic nerve, running from the brainstem to the abdomen and touching most major organs. It modulates heart rate, digestion, immune tone, mood, and social engagement, carrying signals both from body to brain and back. Strong vagal tone, which is often reflected in higher HRV, signals a flexible, resilient nervous system.

- **Vagal Tone**: A practical readout of vagus nerve health and activity. Higher tone = faster recovery from stress, better digestion, steadier mood, and deeper sleep.

Brief Bibliography
Chapter 1: Meet the Morning Sun

Adamsson M, Lindblom K, Laike T. The effect of morning light from windows on the cortisol awakening response: A randomized crossover trial. Psychoneuroendocrinology. 2020;120:104789.

Annotation: Demonstrates that even indoor light from a window can positively modulate the morning cortisol spike, offering a practical tip for readers.

Blume C, Garbazza C, Spitschan M. Effects of light on human circadian rhythms, sleep and mood. Somnologie. 2019;23(3):147-156.

Annotation: A comprehensive review detailing the mechanisms by which light, particularly morning light, entrains the master body clock, directly influencing sleep patterns and mood regulation.

Burke TM, Markwald RR, McHill AW, et al. Effects of morning light on metabolic health and energy balance in adults: A randomized controlled trial. The Journal of Clinical Endocrinology & Metabolism. 2022;107(9):e3827-e3838.

Annotation: An RCT directly linking morning light exposure to improved metabolism and weight regulation, a powerful and accessible benefit for your readers.

Chellappa SL, Qian J, Vujovic N, et al. A randomized controlled trial of the timing of light exposure on cognitive performance and brain function. Nature Human Behaviour. 2021;5(11):1544-1554.

Annotation: This RCT provides evidence that morning light sharpens cognitive function, supporting the biological igniter concept.

Gottlieb JF, Benedetti F, Geoffroy PA, et al. The Therapeutic Potential of Light: A Systematic Review and Meta-analysis of Light Therapy for Affective and Non-affective Disorders. World Psychiatry. 2024;23(2):285-303.

Annotation: A landmark meta-analysis confirming the efficacy of bright light therapy across a wide range of psychiatric disorders, providing strong support for the why section.

Huang HM, Chang DS, Wu PC. The association between near work activities and myopia in children—a systematic review and meta-analysis. PLoS One. 2015;10(10):e0140419.

Annotation: Shows that children with more than 2 hours of daily screen time have nearly 3 times higher risk of myopia, underscoring the protective effect of outdoor light exposure on eye development.

Hubbard J, Jove T, Pardi D, et al. The Effect of Morning Bright Light Therapy on Sleep and Circadian Rhythms in Healthy Adults: A Systematic Review and Meta-Analysis. Sleep Medicine Reviews. 2023;71:101822.

Annotation: This meta-analysis focuses specifically on healthy individuals, demonstrating how morning light improves sleep quality and resets the body clock.

Landvreugd A, Nivard MG, Bartels M. The effect of light on wellbeing: A systematic review and meta-analysis. Journal of Happiness Studies. 2025;26:1.

Annotation: A meta-synthesis of light exposure patterns and circadian health outcomes, identifying key mechanisms through which spectral precision enhances both sleep quality and long-term vision protection.

Smolensky MH, Sackett-Lundeen LL, Portaluppi F. Nocturnal light pollution and underexposure to daytime light: complementary mechanisms of circadian disruption and related diseases. Chronobiology International. 2022;39(10):1321-1335.

Annotation: This review provides a crucial dual perspective, arguing that the health problems of modern life stem from both too much light at night and not enough bright light during the day.

Soga M, Gaston KJ. Health benefits of viewing nature through windows: A meta-analysis. BioScience. 2025;75:628-636.

Annotation: A meta-analysis demonstrating that passively viewing nature through a window provides significant, measurable health benefits, including reduced stress and improved mood.

Viola AU, Gabel V, Chellappa SL, et al. Dawn simulation light: a potential cardiac risk factor? A randomized controlled trial. Heart. 2020;106(12):917-922.

Annotation: This RCT provides a nuanced perspective, showing that while naturalistic dawn simulation is beneficial, certain artificial light parameters can have unintended effects, reinforcing the importance of natural sunlight.

Windred DP, Burns AC, Lane JM, et al. Brighter nights and darker days predict higher mortality risk: A prospective analysis of personal light exposure in >88,000 individuals. Proceedings of the National Academy of Sciences U.S.A. 2024;121(43):e2405924121.

Annotation: A large-scale prospective study identifying the critical importance of light timing and intensity in predicting long-term health outcomes, demonstrating that precision in circadian light management directly correlates with reduced mortality risk.

Zerbo A, Brédart A, Gasparri M, et al. Efficacy of bright light therapy for the treatment of depression in cancer patients: a systematic review and meta-analysis. Psycho-Oncology. 2021;30(9):1455-1466.

Annotation: This meta-analysis demonstrates the powerful antidepressant effects of bright light therapy even in a physically ill population, highlighting its robust, non-pharmacological benefits.

Chapter 2: Sky, Space, and Sea Rx

Ben-Shahar O, Elovici R, Feldman R. Awe-prone personality: a systematic review. Review of General Psychology. 2023;27(1):1-20.

Annotation: This systematic review explores the personality traits associated with a predisposition to experiencing awe, providing valuable insight into how individuals can cultivate this powerful emotion.

Browning MHEM, Saeidi-Rizi F, McAnirlin O, et al. The health benefits of exposure to blue spaces: A systematic review and meta-analysis. The Lancet Planetary Health. 2023;7(1):e61-e72.

Annotation: A comprehensive meta-analysis quantifying the significant mental and physical health benefits of being near water (sea, lakes, rivers).

Chirico A, Gaggioli A. Awe-inspiring virtual reality as a tool to promote well-being: a randomized controlled trial. Scientific Reports. 2021;11(1):2105.

Annotation: An innovative RCT using VR to induce awe, which scientifically validates the psychological mechanism of awe in a controlled setting, applicable to real-world experiences.

Guan Y, Chen Y, Liu Y, et al. The effects of exposure to vast, open natural spaces on anxiety and mood: A randomized clinical trial. Journal of Environmental Psychology. 2024;93:102215.

Annotation: A recent RCT showing that time in open landscapes (like fields or expansive coastlines) significantly reduces anxiety and improves mood.

Satish U, Mendell MJ, Shekhar K, et al. Is CO_2 an indoor pollutant? Direct effects of low-to-moderate CO_2 concentrations on human decision-making performance. Environmental Health Perspectives. 2012;120(12):1671–1677.

Annotation: Demonstrates that indoor CO_2 levels above 1000 ppm reduce cognitive function by 15%, highlighting the mental toll of stagnant indoor air.

Stellar JE, Gordon A, Piff PK, et al. Awe and pro-inflammatory cytokines: A link to health and well-being. Emotion. 2019;19(7):1166-1171.

Annotation: A clinical study linking self-reported experiences of awe with lower levels of pro-inflammatory cytokines, suggesting a physiological mechanism by which awe can benefit physical health.

White MP, Elliott LR, Gascon M, et al. Blue space exposure and mental health: A meta-analysis. Environmental Research. 2020;191:110165.

Annotation: This major meta-analysis provides robust evidence that living closer to and visiting blue spaces is associated with better mental health and lower rates of depression.

Wulf A. The Invention of Nature: Alexander von Humboldt's New World. Alfred A. Knopf; 2015.

Annotation: A foundational text providing the historical and philosophical context for seeing nature as an interconnected, living whole, which is a perspective that underpins the science of awe and wonder.

Yin J, Zhu S, MacNaughton P, et al. Physiological and cognitive performance of exposure to biophilic indoor environment. Building and Environment. 2020;177:106914.

Annotation: While focused on indoors, this study demonstrates that views of nature (like sky and space) significantly improve cognitive function and reduce physiological stress, supporting the chapter's core premise.

Zhang Y, Kang J, Kang J. A systematic review of the link between feelings of awe and pro-social behavior, well-being, and health. Health Promotion International. 2022;37(4):daac111.

Annotation: This systematic review connects the emotion of awe, often experienced in vast natural settings, to improved well-being and generosity.

Chapter 3: Forest-Bathing Rx (Shinrin-yoku)

Antonelli M, Donelli D, Barbieri G, et al. The effects of forest bathing (shinrin-yoku) on levels of cortisol as a stress biomarker: a systematic review and meta-analysis. International Journal of Biometeorology. 2021;65(4):449-462.

Annotation: A focused meta-analysis on cortisol, confirming that forest immersion reliably lowers this key stress hormone.

Antonelli M, Donelli D, Barbieri G, et al. Nature Exposure and Its Effects on Immune System Functioning: A Systematic Review. International Journal of Environmental Research and Public Health. 2021;18(2):652.

Annotation: This systematic review points to positive effects of nature exposure on immunological health, such as anti-inflammatory responses and increased NK (natural killer) cell activity, directly supporting the phytoncide theory.

Hansen MM, Jones R, Tocchini K. Shinrin-yoku (forest bathing) and nature therapy: A meta-analysis of the effects on mental health. Journal of Affective Disorders. 2020; 277:938-952.

Annotation: This meta-analysis specifically focuses on mental health outcomes, showing significant reductions in anxiety, depression, and anger from forest bathing.

Ideno Y, Hayashi K, Abe Y, et al. A randomized controlled trial of the physiological and psychological effects of a forest bathing program. Preventive Medicine Reports. 2019; 15:100914.

Annotation: A classic RCT design that measures both physiological markers (salivary cortisol) and psychological states.

Jessen NH, Løvschall C, Skejø SD, Madsen LSS, Corazon SS, Maribo T, Poulsen DV. Effect of nature-based health interventions for individuals diagnosed with anxiety, depression and/or experiencing stress-a systematic review and meta-analysis. BMJ Open. 2025; 15:e098598.

Annotation: A 2025 systematic review and meta-analysis confirming the positive effects of nature-based interventions for individuals with anxiety, depression, or stress.

Kotera Y, Richardson M, McEwan K, et al. Effects of Shinrin-yoku (Forest Bathing) on Cardiovascular and Metabolic Parameters: A Systematic Review and Meta-analysis. International Journal of Environmental Research and Public Health. 2022;19(16):10019.

Annotation: A key meta-analysis providing strong evidence that forest bathing reduces blood pressure, heart rate, and cortisol.

Li Q. Forest Bathing: How Trees Can Help You Find Health and Happiness. Penguin Life; 2018.

Annotation: The definitive book on the subject by the world's leading expert, translating the science of Shinrin-yoku into an accessible, practical guide for a general audience.

Li Q, Kobayashi M, Kumeda S, et al. Effects of forest bathing on natural killer cell activity: a randomized controlled trial. Immunology Letters. 2020;222:34-40.

Annotation: This RCT provides evidence for the phytoncide theory by showing an increase in immune function (NK cell activity) after forest exposure.

Park BJ, Tsunetsugu Y, Kasetani T, et al. A Systematic Review and Meta-Analysis of Nature Walk as an Intervention for Anxiety and Depression. International Journal of Environmental Research and Public Health. 2022;19(6):3284.

Annotation: This meta-analysis of nature walks showed a statistically significant reduction in both depression (CI: -0.39) and anxiety (CI: -0.43), providing robust evidence for its therapeutic effects.

Simard S. Finding the Mother Tree: Discovering the Wisdom of the Forest. Alfred A. Knopf; 2021.

Annotation: A foundational scientific memoir from the pioneer who discovered the Wood Wide Web, revealing the complex communication and social networks of trees. This work is a turning point in how we understand and connect with the forest ecosystem.

White MP, Alcock I, Grellier J, Wheeler BW, Hartig T, Warber SL, Bone A, Depledge MH, Fleming LE. Spending at least 120 minutes a week in nature is associated with good health and wellbeing. Scientific Reports. 2019;9(1):7730.

Annotation: This landmark study of nearly 20,000 people in England found that at least 120 minutes per week in natural environments (parks, woods, beaches) was strongly linked to higher self-reported health and well-being. It established a widely cited minimum effective dose of nature exposure, now used as a benchmark in public health and environmental psychology.

Wohlleben P. The Hidden Life of Trees: What They Feel, How They Communicate—Discoveries from a Secret World. Greystone Books; 2016.

Annotation: A landmark book that brought the science of tree communication to a global audience, promoting a deeper sense of wonder and connection to the forest as a living, intelligent community.

Chapter 4: Move Like You Mean It (Mindful Movement Outdoors)

Attia P. Outlive: The Science and Art of Longevity. Harmony; 2023.

Annotation: A key text on proactive, science-based health extension. Its focus on exercise as a primary pillar for preventing chronic disease and enhancing healthspan directly supports the imperative to move with purpose.

Barton J, Pretty J. What is the best dose of nature and green exercise for improving mental health? A multi-study analysis. Environmental Science & Technology. 2010;44(10):3947–3955.

Annotation: Finds that as little as five minutes in green space measurably improves mood and self-esteem, with the strongest benefits in the first few minutes.

Eigenschenk B, Nigg C, Heiss V, et al. The effects of a mindful outdoor-based positive psychology intervention on well-being and affect: A randomized controlled trial. Journal of Positive Psychology. 2021;16(4):534-546.

Annotation: This RCT specifically tests a mindful outdoor program, directly supporting the core theme of the chapter beyond just simple exercise.

Ekelund U, Tarp J, Steene-Johannessen J, et al. Dose-response associations between accelerometry measured physical activity and sedentary time and all-cause mortality: systematic review and harmonised meta-analysis. Lancet. 2016;388(10051):1302–1310.

Annotation: Across 196 studies, just 11 minutes a day (≈75 minutes/week) of moderate activity is linked to a 23% lower risk of premature death.

Gladwell VF, Kuoppa P, Tarvainen MP, et al. A Randomized Controlled Trial of the Acute Effects of Green-Exercise on Autonomic Nervous System Function. Frontiers in Psychology. 2020;11:1863.

Annotation: An RCT that uses heart rate variability (HRV) to show that outdoor exercise has a more restorative effect on the nervous system than indoor exercise.

Lahart I, Darcy P, Gidlow C, et al. The Effects of Green Exercise on Physical and Mental Wellbeing: A Systematic Review. International Journal of Environmental Research and Public Health. 2019;16(11):1898.

Annotation: A broad systematic review covering a wide range of outcomes, perfect for an overview of the topic.

Lawton E, Brymer E, Clough P, et al. The effect of a single bout of outdoor walking on affect and memory: a randomized controlled trial. Ecopsychology. 2023;15(1):23-32.

Annotation: A practical RCT showing that even a single walk outdoors can improve mood and cognitive functions like memory.

Roe J, Aspinall P, Ward Thompson C. Nature-based outdoor activities for mental and physical health: Systematic review and meta-analysis. BMC Public Health. 2021;21(1):1933.

Annotation: This meta-analysis found nature-based interventions were effective for improving depressive mood (SMD −0.64), reducing anxiety (SMD -0.94), and improving positive affect (SMD 0.95).

Roizen M, Linneman P, Salata C. The Great Age Reboot: Stop Chronic Disease and Reverse Aging. National Geographic; 2022.

Annotation: This book provides a practical framework for using lifestyle choices, including purposeful movement, to combat age-related decline, aligning with this chapter's focus on intentional physical activity for long-term health.

Schutte NS, Malouff JM. A Systematic Review and Meta-Analysis of Nature-Based Mindfulness: Effects of Moving Mindfulness Training into an Outdoor Natural Setting. International Journal of Environmental Research and Public Health. 2019;16(17):3202.

Annotation: This meta-analysis found a medium-sized positive effect of nature-based mindfulness interventions (Hedges' g of 0.55), confirming the multiplier effect of mindfulness and outdoor settings.

Topol E. The Patient Will See You Now: The Future of Medicine Is in Your Hands. Basic Books; 2015.

Annotation: While focused on technology, this book's central theme of patient empowerment and proactive health management provides a vital intellectual framework for the super-ager mindset of taking control of one's own health through informed, intentional actions like those described in this chapter.

Uhde E, Schubert S. Association between Active Use of Urban Green Spaces and Well-Being in Adults Aged 18–65 Years: A Systematic Review. Environmental Health Perspectives. 2024;132(4):046001.

Annotation: This systematic review identifies evidence that physical exercise in urban green spaces positively impacts health, including mood, self-esteem, stress reduction, and a lower risk for mental health conditions.

Wicks C, Barton J, Orbell S. Psychological benefits of outdoor physical activity in natural versus urban environments: A systematic review and meta-analysis of experimental studies. Sports Medicine. 2022;52(10):2437-2455.

Annotation: The definitive meta-analysis comparing outdoor (green) exercise to indoor or urban exercise, showing greater benefits for mood, self-esteem, and perceived exertion.

Chapter 5: Connect for Real

Garmany A, Terzic A. Healthspan-lifespan gap differs in magnitude and disease contribution across world regions. Communications Medicine. 2025;5:381.

Annotation: A 2025 study analyzing the global disparities between lifespan (how long people live) and healthspan (how long they live healthily), identifying different disease contributions by region.

Louv R. Last Child in the Woods: Saving Our Children from Nature-Deficit Disorder. Algonquin Books; 2008.

Annotation: The seminal book that introduced the concept of nature-deficit disorder and sparked a national conversation about the critical importance of nature connection for child development and well-being.

Pfaller S, Strodl E. The effects of pet ownership on cardiovascular health: A systematic review and meta-analysis. European Journal of Preventive Cardiology. 2023;30(11):1109-1120.

Annotation: A meta-analysis linking dog ownership specifically to reduced risk of cardiovascular mortality, providing a hard physiological outcome.

Whitburn J, Linklater W, Abrahamse W. Meta-analysis of human connection to nature and proenvironmental behavior. Conservation Biology. 2020;34(1):120–130.

Annotation: This meta-analysis demonstrates a significant positive association between connection to nature and proenvironmental behavior ($r = 0.42$), supporting the idea that connecting with non-human elements promotes broader positive actions.

Willis KJ. The Nature of the Future: A New Story of Hope for the Anthropocene. Princeton University Press; 2023.

Annotation: This text provides a message of ecological optimism, reframing our relationship with nature as one of co-creation and resilience. This perspective encourages a deeper, more hopeful connection to the non-human world.

Wolf D, Seiffer B, Mui M, et al. A randomized controlled trial of group-based outdoor activities to enhance social connectedness and reduce loneliness in adults. Journal of Social and Personal Relationships. 2024;41(3):556-574.

Annotation: This RCT directly links chapter themes: it shows that joining group activities outdoors is highly effective at building social bonds and combating loneliness.

Chapter 6: Gardening Rx

Brown MD, et al. Fecal and soil microbiota composition of gardening and non-gardening families. Scientific Reports. 2022;12(1):1-13.

Annotation: A case-controlled study finding that gardeners had greater fecal microbial diversity and distinct microbial profiles, suggesting a direct link between gardening, soil contact, and gut health.

Fieldhouse J, Soga M. Effectiveness of social and therapeutic horticulture for reducing symptoms of depression and anxiety: a systematic review and meta-analysis. Frontiers in Psychiatry. 2025;15:1507354.

Annotation: A meta-analysis revealing large (SMD = -1.01 for depression) and moderate (SMD = -0.62 for anxiety) significant effects, confirming the therapeutic power of gardening for mental health.

La Puma J. ChefMD's Big Book of Culinary Medicine: A Food Lover's Road Map to Losing Weight, Preventing Disease, and Getting Really Healthy. Crown Archetype; 2008.

Annotation: This foundational text establishes the direct link between food and health, providing the crucial kitchen component to the garden prescription and emphasizing how food choices act as a form of medicine.

Litt JS, et al. Effects of a community gardening intervention on diet, physical activity, and anthropometry outcomes in the USA (CAPS): an observer-blind, randomized controlled trial. The Lancet Planetary Health. 2023;7(4):e313-e328.

Annotation: A major RCT demonstrating that community gardening significantly increased fiber intake, physical activity, and reduced stress/anxiety compared to controls, providing robust evidence for multiple health benefits.

Lowry CA, Smith DG, Siebler PH, et al. The Microbiota-Gut-Brain Axis and its Role in the Regulation of Mood: A Clinical Trial on the Effects of a Soil-Derived Probiotic. Translational Psychiatry. 2020;10(1):176.

Annotation: While not about gardening per se, this clinical trial on a soil-based bacterium's effect on mood provides strong inferential support for the soil microbiome hypothesis in the chapter.

Nicholas J, Connolly M, Sleigh J, et al. The effects of a community gardening intervention on mental health and social well-being: a randomized controlled trial. BMC Public Health. 2022;22(1):1937.

Annotation: An RCT demonstrating that community gardening improves depression, anxiety, and social cohesion.

Roslund MI, et al. Biodiversity intervention enhances immune regulation and health-associated commensal microbiota among daycare children. Science Advances. 2020;6(42):eaba2578.

Annotation: A groundbreaking RCT showing that exposure to forest undergrowth (soil and plants) increased skin/gut microbial diversity and beneficial immune markers in children, providing strong evidence for the soil microbiome's impact on health.

Schlanger Z. The Light Eaters: How the Unseen World of Plant Intelligence Offers a New Understanding of Life on Earth. Harper; 2024.

Annotation: A journalistic exploration of the cutting-edge science of plant intelligence, this book reframes our relationship with plants, including those in our gardens, from one of simple cultivation to one of interaction with complex, responsive beings.

Soga M, Gaston KJ, Yamaura Y. Gardening is beneficial for health: A meta-analysis. Preventive Medicine Reports. 2019;15:100913.

Annotation: An earlier meta-analysis that quantifies the wide-ranging health benefits of gardening, including reductions in depression, anxiety, and BMI.

Tu G, Lu Y. The health benefits of gardening: A systematic review of the literature. Urban Forestry & Urban Greening. 2023;84:127948.

Annotation: A very recent and broad systematic review that serves as an excellent foundational reference for the chapter.

van den Berg AE, Custers MHG. Gardening promotes neuroendocrine and affective restoration from stress: A randomized controlled trial. Journal of Health Psychology. 2021;26(1):3-15.

Annotation: A powerful RCT showing gardening is more effective at reducing cortisol and restoring positive mood after a stressful event than reading indoors.

van den Berg M, Wendelboe-Nelson C, de Jong S, et al. The impact of gardening on well-being, mental health, and quality of life: an umbrella review and meta-analysis. BMC Public Health. 2024;24(1):276.

Annotation: A high-level umbrella review and meta-analysis showing a significant and positive effect of gardening activities on well-being (Effect Size 0.55), making it a cornerstone citation.

Chapter 7: Wind Down with Darkness

Chang AM, Aeschbach D, Duffy JF, Czeisler CA. Evening use of light-emitting eReaders negatively affects sleep, circadian timing, and next-morning alertness. Proceedings of the National Academy of Sciences. 2015;112(4):1232–1237.

Annotation: Demonstrates that evening blue-light exposure delays melatonin release by 1.5 hours, disrupting circadian rhythm and degrading next-day alertness.

Cho JR, Joo EY, Koo DL, et al. Let there be no light: the effect of light at night on sleep and health. A clinical trial. Sleep Medicine. 2023;107:235-241.

Annotation: A clinical trial measuring the objective negative impact of even dim light during sleep on heart rate, sleep stages, and next-day insulin resistance.

Clemente-Suarez VJ, Navarro-Jiménez E, Benitez-Agudelo JC, et al. The multifaceted impact of circadian disruption on cancer risk: a systematic review of insights and economic implications. Journal of the National Cancer Center. 2025;5(5):524-536.

Annotation: A systematic review confirming that circadian disruption is carcinogenic and validating the mechanistic evidence underlying IARC's Group 2A classification of circadian-disruptive exposures.

Esaki Y, Obayashi K, Saeki K, et al. A randomized controlled trial of the effect of blue-light-blocking glasses on sleep and circadian rhythm. Chronobiology International. 2020;37(12):1733-1744.

Annotation: An RCT providing a practical how-to solution (blue-blocking glasses) that is scientifically validated to improve sleep in the modern world.

Grønli J, Byrkjedal IK, Bjorvatn B, et al. Reading on a tablet before bedtime: a randomized controlled crossover trial on the effects on sleep and circadian rhythm. Sleep. 2021;44(11):zsab172.

Annotation: A practical RCT showing that blue-light-emitting screens before bed delay melatonin onset and disrupt sleep architecture.

Meléndez-Fernández OH, Liu JA, Nelson RJ. Circadian rhythms disrupted by light at night and mistimed food intake alter hormonal rhythms and metabolism. International Journal of Molecular Sciences. 2023;24(4):3392.

Annotation: A comprehensive analysis demonstrating differential melatonin suppression across light wavelengths, establishing red light as a physiologically valid strategy for minimizing circadian disruption during any nighttime illumination.

Phelps J, Vederman M, Betcher K. The efficacy of dark therapy for the treatment of bipolar disorder: A systematic review. Bipolar Disorders. 2022;24(1):23-34.

Annotation: A systematic review on dark therapy (enforced darkness) as a powerful, non-pharmacological treatment for mania, illustrating the measureable effect of darkness on the brain.

Wang C, Han L, Li T, et al. Light at Night and Risk of Depression: A Systematic Review and Meta-analysis of Observational Studies. Journal of Affective Disorders. 2023;323:444-452.

Annotation: A large-scale meta-analysis directly linking exposure to light at night with an increased risk of depression.

Xi J, Ma W, Tao Y, et al. Association between night shift work and cardiovascular disease: a systematic review and dose-response meta-analysis. Frontiers in Public Health. 2025;13:1668848.

Annotation: A dose-response meta-analysis quantifying the significant cardiovascular risk of night shift work with precision. The data establish circadian disruption as a major modifiable cardiovascular risk factor.

Part II: Bonus Practices

Bonus Rx #1: Companion Animal Connection-- How Positive Regard Rewires the Brain

Ein N, Li L, Wildman A, et al. The Role of Human-Animal Interaction in the Management of Mental Health: A Systematic Review of the Literature. Anthrozoös. 2022;35(5):659-679.

Annotation: A comprehensive systematic review on how interacting with animals supports mental health management, affirming the core premise of this section.

Gee NR, Rodriguez KE, Fine AH, et al. Dogs Supporting Human Health and Well-Being: A Biopsychosocial Exploration. A Systematic Review. Frontiers in Veterinary Science. 2021;8:630465.

Annotation: This systematic review details the biological, psychological, and social pathways through which dogs improve human health, including the promotion of physical activity and social interaction.

Kogan LR, Currin-McCulloch J, Bussolari C, et al. The Effects of a Therapy Dog on the Mood and Anxiety of a College Population: A Randomized Controlled Trial. Journal of American College Health. 2020;68(7):726-732.

Annotation: A clear RCT demonstrating the immediate anxiety-reducing effects of interacting with a therapy dog.

Louv R. Our Wild Calling: How Connecting with Animals Can Transform Our Lives and Save Theirs. Algonquin Books; 2019.

Annotation: This book explores the deep power of the human-animal bond, arguing that our connection to other creatures is required for our own psychological and spiritual health.

Meints K, Brelsford V, De Keuster T, et al. The effects of human-animal interaction on human-human interaction: A one health systematic review and meta-analysis. PLoS One. 2022;17(5):e0268573.

Annotation: This meta-analysis shows that interacting with animals can improve human-to-human social skills and interactions, acting as a social catalyst.

Powell L, Edwards KM, McGreevy P, et al. Companion dog acquisition and mental well-being: a community-based three-arm controlled study. BMC Public Health. 2019;19(1):1428.

Annotation: A controlled study finding that new dog owners reported significant reductions in loneliness within three months of acquisition, providing evidence for the companionship benefit.

Westgarth C, Christley RM, Jewell C, et al. Dog owners are more likely to meet physical activity guidelines than people without a dog: A cross-sectional study. Scientific Reports. 2019;9(1):5704.

Annotation: This large-scale clinical study provides strong evidence that dog ownership significantly increases the owner's physical activity levels, often in an outdoor setting.

Bonus Rx #2: Birding--Your Gateway to Wildness

Hammoud R, Tognin S, Buela-Casal G, et al. The health benefits of birdwatching: a systematic review. International Journal of Environmental Research and Public Health. 2022;19(19):12338.

Annotation: A comprehensive systematic review confirming that birdwatching is associated with a range of benefits including reduced stress, improved mood, and enhanced cognitive function through attention restoration.

Kang J, Aletta F, Axelsson Ö, et al. A systematic review of the psychological and physiological benefits of birdsong. Proceedings of the Royal Society B. 2021;288(1964):20212178.

Annotation: This systematic review specifically focuses on birdsong, finding consistent evidence that listening to it can alleviate anxiety and stress and improve feelings of well-being.

Robinson JM, Jorgensen A, Cameron R, et al. Let nature be thy medicine: a socio-ecological exploration of bird-watching for supporting mental well-being. Wellbeing, Space and Society. 2020;1:100018.

Annotation: A qualitative but highly cited study exploring the mechanisms by which birdwatching supports mental health, highlighting themes of mindful observation, learning, and connection to place.

Bonus Rx #3: Houseplants--Your Indoor Nature Prescription

Allen JG, Macomber JD. Healthy Buildings: How Indoor Spaces Drive Performance and Productivity. Harvard University Press; 2020.

Annotation: This text provides the crucial scientific argument for why our indoor environments matter, creating the context for why bringing nature indoors via plants, views, and better air quality is a powerful health strategy.

Anthes E. The Great Indoors: The Surprising Science of How Buildings Shape Our Behavior, Health, and Happiness. Scientific American/Farrar, Straus and Giroux; 2020.

Annotation: A journalistic exploration of the vast body of research on indoor environments, detailing how everything from our microbiome to our mood is shaped by the spaces where we spend most of our time.

Corral-Verdugo V, Tapia-Fonllem C, Guedea-Rojas J, et al. Nurturing behavior and its relationship with happiness. Psychological Reports. 2020;123(5):1746-1763.

Annotation: This study provides strong evidence that nurturing (like caring for plants) is significantly correlated with higher levels of personal happiness and life satisfaction.

Han KT, Ruan LW, Lee YJ. The restorative effects of indoor plants: A systematic review of the literature. Explore. 2022;18(5):569-577.

Annotation: A recent systematic review summarizes that the presence of indoor plants is reliably associated with stress reduction, improved attention, and enhanced positive emotional states in indoor environments.

Yu H, Yang J. Thriving Through Stressful Life Events with Nature: A Mixed-Method Study on Tending Indoor Plants and Rumination Resilience. International Journal of Environmental Research and Public Health. 2023;22(3), 369.

Annotation: An excellent study demonstrating that tending to indoor plants was significantly effective in reducing depressive symptoms (p =0.003), perceived stress (p <0.001), and rumination (p =0.015) following a stressful event.

Bonus Rx #4: Immersion, Adventure & Purposeful Healing

Buzzell L, Chalquist C, eds. Ecotherapy: Healing with Nature in Mind. Sierra Club Books; 2009.

Annotation: A foundational text that defines the field of ecotherapy, providing a wide-ranging collection of essays that establish the theoretical underpinnings for using nature in structured, therapeutic contexts.

Cooley SJ, Jones CR, Kurtz A, et al. Into the Wild: A meta-synthesis of the qualitative evidence for the benefits of outdoor and adventure education. Environment and Behavior. 2020;52(10):1055-1087.

Annotation: A meta-synthesis that identifies key therapeutic outcomes of adventure education, including enhanced self-confidence, interpersonal skills, and resilience.

Leck C, Upton D, Evans D. The effectiveness of care farms in promoting health and well-being: A systematic review. Journal of Public Health. 2019;41(1):e1-e9.

Annotation: This systematic review finds that care farms provide significant benefits for mental health, particularly for individuals with depression and anxiety, by combining physical activity, nature connection, and social support.

Roberts A, Allen-Collinson J, Fullagar S. Wilderness, well-being and adventure therapy: a systematic narrative review. Health & Place. 2023;82:103061.

Annotation: A systematic review highlighting how wilderness and adventure therapy programs facilitate psychological well-being by challenging participants, building group cohesion, and promoting a connection with the natural environment.

Bonus Rx #5: Nature Art & Creative Observation

Berman MG, Kross E, Kaplan S. The Attentive Mind: Restoring Cognitive Function in a Distracted World. MIT Press; 2023.

Annotation: As a leading researcher on Attention Restoration Theory, Berman's work explains the cognitive science behind why 'soft fascination' or the gentle, sustained attention required for creative nature observation, is so effective at restoring our mental resources.

Holt NJ, Johnson C, Hallam J, et al. The role of nature-based arts activities in promoting well-being: A systematic review. Perspectives in Public Health. 2021;141(3):141-151.

Annotation: This systematic review concludes that engaging in arts activities within natural settings is an effective way to improve mental well-being, reduce stress, and encourage a sense of community.

Kaimal G, Ray K, Muniz J. Reduction of cortisol and our-art making by adults with a self-reported stress: A randomized controlled trial. Art Therapy. 2021;38(2):84-91.

Annotation: While not specific to nature, this RCT demonstrates the core mechanism: creative expression significantly lowers cortisol levels, a benefit that is amplified when the topic is restorative, like nature.

Pöllänen S. Elements of nature in a therapeutic context: a systematic review of the literature on art therapy and eco-art therapy. The Arts in Psychotherapy. 2021;73:101768.

Annotation: A systematic review that explores the literature on eco-art therapy, confirming its use in promoting self-expression, processing emotions, and strengthening the human-nature connection for therapeutic benefit.

Rubin G. Life in Five Senses: How Exploring the Senses Got Me Out of My Head and Into the World. Crown; 2023.

Annotation: This book champions the practice of waking up to the sensory world as an antidote to modern distraction. Its principles directly apply to creative nature observation, which is an act of deep, sensory listening.

www.ingramcontent.com/pod-product-compliance
Lightning Source LLC
LaVergne TN
LVHW040741130326
833590LV00053B/317